Lose The Fat: Without The Exercise

By

William Thrash

Self-Help Guides
By William Thrash

You Are In Control

Novels

MANSION – *A Horror Novel*
The Goblin Adventure – *A Fantasy*

Novellas

Winning Hands – *A Western*
The Dwarven Legacy – *A Fantasy*
The Melaki Chronicle – *A Fantasy*
DRAGON, RAMPANT – *A Novel*
The Melaki Chronicle Volume II – *A Fantasy*
Tuesdays – *A Modern Horror*
Duke Kord Becker – *A Fantasy*
Eliam Cross: Swords & Treachery – *A Fantasy*

Cover Photo by Shutterstock.com

**"When your diet is wrong, medicine is of no use.
When your diet is correct, medicine is of no need"**
Ayurvedic Proverb

Introduction

There's a difference between old and new, out-of-date and cutting edge, and wrong information and right.

This is a booklet on food and how the body reacts to various factors of food intake and environment. In it, I approach information in an unconventional way. Most books on diet are written by someone who first went to college, studied the textbook of someone else's opinion, and then walked away with a degree.

I did not. In fact, I boast of not having a degree in nutrition. Why? A degree is a proclamation to all that the bearer has passed a specific curriculum of learning in a set of information that may very well now be outdated. Take a fictional young man who earns that degree. He graduated last week, ready to aid those in need of nutritional advice. He knows what there is to know from being taught. Yesterday, a new study breaks onto the scene that directly contradicts the five or six year old information (or older) he believes is the rock-solid truth. Is he right in proclaiming the old information just because he has a Master's?

To illustrate, I got into a small argument with one nutritional "expert" who had a Master's. He proclaimed soy was the absolute healthiest food on the planet and he was an expert with a Master's Degree and knew what he was talking about. I asked him how he could view the world's most powerful source of inflammation as anything but unhealthy and he went silent. That was the end of the conversation, except that he called me names and rested on his degree. Think about this, though, do we need a Master's to understand something?

Do you need to be a biologist to know drinking battery acid is bad?

Do you need to be a marine biologist to know fish come from the water?

Do you need to be an astrologer to know when the moon is full?

Do you need to be an astronomer to know the sun rises in the east?

You see, I wasn't relying on someone else's opinion from a textbook – or old information, if you will. I was relying on the most recent studies I could get my hands on. That Master's holder probably learned about soy before all the medical studies came out that showed how horrible it is in causing inflammation in the body.

The point is, some things can be deduced from reasoned consideration and you don't need a college diploma specifically dealing with that area to have an informed opinion.

But before any might think I claim some enlightened intelligence; I do not. I repeat what I hear from doctors, chemists, biologists – those sounding the alarm that things aren't right. I simply apply my intellect to reasoning what they say, peruse their quoted studies, and consider the evidence at hand. Much like a judge. No judge is an expert at anything except being a judge. Yet they often decide the truth of the matter as the evidence is presented. I only ask that we all act as our own judges on what we face daily.

So the approach here with the information in this booklet will be with the most current research available. Please note that new research may very well invalidate parts of this information in the coming years.

However, the dietary effects, the environmental factors, and the plan of losing fat *without exercise* as presented in this book work. Which means, the foods, conditions and strategies listed here have been shown to work and will likely not be invalidated as wrong. There may be better ways researched in months or years ahead - faster, more efficient. Conversely, new foods might be introduced that pervert the foods listed here: the big danger is unlabeled genetically modified food. However, if the reader can follow this booklet's simple food recommendations and be sure of how this food was grown/produced, losing fat should be about as easy as packing on all that weight to begin with.

Easy? Yes, easy. Read my lips. Easy. E-Z. All it takes is time as your body shifts back into healthy digestion and begins utilizing stored fat. No exercise is required, though some minor exercise won't hurt. Strenuous exercise should be strictly avoided. More on why later.

No enormous amounts of willpower are required. You do not need the mental strength of a Zen Master to turn your body back into a fat-burning machine. In hindsight, you will find it easy. Initially, you may find your body resisting the desire to switch your diet from fat-adding foods to fat-burning foods. That's your body's addiction to the chemicals. Also, you may find the short menu of "safe" foods to be limited. Unfortunately, there isn't much that can be done about that until more organic farms begin producing more organic choices.

Is this book all about organics? No, not really. There is far more to what is making us fat and how to lose it than whether or not a farmer uses petroleum fertilizers or horse manure. There are environmental factors to consider. There are nutritional factors to consider. One hot dog is not the same as the next. All hand sanitizers are not equal. Skin lotions are not all identical.

My food menu presented here will likely expand in the months and years ahead. New studies will undoubtedly expose even more environmental factors that are making us fat. Using what you find in this booklet will most definitely cause a change in direction from fatter and fatter to leaner and leaner and will continue to do so. I suggest we all keep our eyes open for new revelations in research that may further aid our quest for losing that fat for good.

There are no gimmicks in this book. No recommendations for the latest unhealthy "fat pill."

I'll say right here that there never will be a "fat pill" that does not otherwise also destroy your health. I do not present the latest fad diet that doesn't work, nor do I push one weird exercise that will make you as thin as a cadaver with just one minute of exercise per week. Neither do I push a fifteen minute strenuous exercise program as "easy" and "simple" that is guaranteed to make you look like a runway model.

Why, when the media is replete with dietary advice, do Westerners keep getting fatter and fatter? Why do we exercise more and more but still pack on pound after pound? Why, no matter how religiously we follow fad diets, do they not work?

You'll find out why. Read on.

CHAPTER 1

Throw out everything you've been taught about nutrition. That's right, throw it out. Consider everything you've learned about nutrition to be wrong (because it probably is). If you've gotten your knowledge from newsstand magazines or talk shows, throw it out and throw it far. The difference between what we're told day after day and the truth is as stark as dark and light.

Everything we have been taught about diet is a lie.

Fat is bad. *No it's not.*

Wheat is good. *No it's not.*

Meat is bad. *No it's not.*

Anything in moderation is good. ***No**, it is not.*

Is a bullet to the head in moderation "good?"

Is rat poison in moderation good?

Is drinking radioactive sludge in moderation good?

Is eating salmonella-tainted shrimp every day in moderation good?

I hate the word "moderation." It is used to excuse the consumption of very toxic and dangerous foods. Bad things, in moderation, are not good. Eating bad things or poisonous things "in moderation" does not make it somehow healthy. No, it is simply bad food and unhealthy, no matter how "moderately" you eat it. Some people throw around the "moderation" label as if to say everything should be consumed and no one better promote avoiding some foods. Eating "in moderation" has not arrested or reversed the avalanche towards obesity that is occurring throughout the West.

"Everything in moderation" is absolutely the worst advice.

Further, there is a popular misconception that no matter what, if you burn more calories than you eat, you will lose weight. *Not true.* Not true, not true, not true. Not all calories are equal[1], though all the "dieticians" will tell you they are. No. No, no, no. Calories are supposed to be measures of energy. But a calorie from soy has a far different effect on the body than a calorie of butter. Depending on the food from which you get that calorie, you could be sweating to the oldies eleven hours per day, burning twice what you took in and not losing the weight you should. In fact, depending on which food that calorie came from, you could gain fat even when you burn more calories than you ate. More on that later.

~ ~ ~

The biggest lie with which I will start is the **Food Pyramid**. All of us were hounded with this in school with colorful pictures and wagging fingers. But it is a lie. There is nothing truthful or legitimate about the Food Pyramid. It was simply a very successful tool to get Westerners eating more carbs – and ever since, no matter how much we exercise, we get fatter. And we are fatter younger. Diabetes, once an "old person's disease," is now striking children before they reach the age of ten[2].

Here is the danger in the Food Pyramid: wheat in the US has been genetically modified since the 1970s. Inserted – not cross-bred, but directly inserted into the genetic structure – was a modified substance that produced uniform stands of wheat and increased the yield in bushels per acre beyond imagination (14 bushels per acre before the GM manipulation, and now around 45 bushels per acre being genetically modified[3]).

The problem is, this substance, gliadin, has been found to be the culprit in a list of maladies longer than the Rio Grande[4]. Allergies, autism, diabetes, Celiac's Disease, irritable bowel syndrome (constipation), etc, etc, ad nauseum.

WHEAT is the one primary immediate substance that must be avoided at all costs. Wheat (typical American wheat) in "moderation" is not good. Is moderate constipation good? Is moderate Celiac's Disease good? Is moderate obesity good? Is moderate diabetes good? Let's look at it this way: we have piled so many unhealthy products into our system that the scales are no longer in balance, they are firmly in the "not registering and failing" arena. To begin to tip the body back to healthiness, we need to be drastic in our pursuit of allowing the body to heal itself. WHEAT is bad. *Avoid*. Skip the bread aisle, entirely. Every single loaf is tainted with genetically modified wheat, soy and canola oils, and thickening gums that cause a host of intestinal maladies (I will address those ingredients later on). However, later, when the body begins to right itself, some wheat is allowable – but only that wheat packaged as organic and non-GMO. It can be found and ordered online.

Mussolini pushed an enormous wheat-planting program in the 1920s in the northern and central areas of Italy[5] - and in the European Union, wheat cannot be genetically modified. So Italian pasta is safe. Be sure, however, to read the ingredients and description. One major Italian pasta maker uses twenty percent American wheat in the mix. Make sure any pasta you buy from Italy is all Italian. But, only when your body has reversed the effects of our wrecked American wheat.

All wheat is bad. Even "whole wheat." Even "multi-grain wheat." Even "seven-grain wheat." Even "all natural" wheat. Avoid it all, completely, totally and don't look back. Not eating bread might seem difficult; gliadin indeed makes it difficult as it acts as an opiate, stimulating craving and addiction[6]. Quitting bread might be the hardest part of this change in your diet. But don't fear, once you turn your body around, there are a couple of non-GMO wheat options.

Consider this: the Food Pyramid – also described as "sound dietary recommendations" – say we should be eating *at least* six to eleven slices of bread per day[7]. I know many overweight people who eat a third of that and are still ballooning up faster than the federal deficit. Eating what the Food

Pyramid requires would make us all four-hundred pound monstrosities requiring scooters to haul our massive butts around. The Food Pyramid's disconnect with reality is insane.

This wheat insanity is just the tip of the iceberg.

CHAPTER 2

The task at hand with foods is so complex and interconnected that it is like picking up one piece of a 2000-piece jigsaw puzzle and attempting to describe the picture. Each bit is going to raise questions and more questions.

But, I'll do my best to be concise.

So far:

Wheat = bad. No-no. Leave it alone. Don't even "cheat" once. No bread, no crackers, no buns, no muffins, no tortillas, no excuses, stop it.

In this bit I want to talk about **STUDIES** first, and then move to **EGGS**. When it comes to studies, disregard everything you read in popular media because most of it is going to be trash. Let me explain. There is no world building established by God or Man where scientists come from the world over to specifically discover things just for the sake of discovering them. In the past, we had individuals who invented things because they had a desire to improve their own lives and those around them. Many of those scientists died penniless. Today, there is a very lucrative industry in science. No scientists employed by universities or corporations for research purposes are going to die broke. But who is paying for studies?

I'll quote here a scientist specifically referring to this very question.

Professor Salman Hyder is talking about the discovery of anti-cancer properties in the flavonoid *apigenin*. "One problem is, because apigenin doesn't have a known specific target in the cancer cell, funding agencies have been reticent to support the research. Also, since apigenin is easily extracted from plants, **pharmaceutical companies don't stand to profit** from the treatment; **hence the industry won't put money into studying something you can grow in your garden**"[8] (Emphasis mine).

The problem is, studies are funded by those looking for something from which they can profit. The lion's share of funding stems directly from industries looking to support their product. An industry official might say to a university researcher, "Here's a million dollars, please identify something in our product that supports heart health." The researchers know that to get continued funding, they better find something that makes their client happy. If, say, the research turns up some very bad news along with "shocking" findings that the garbage actually does some good, the bad news will be ignored. When the soy industry puts out the claim that soy is the world's best food ever, they're ignoring all the rest of the studies that show extremely detrimental effects on the human system. Why would they want to quote the bad?

So when you see a new study pushed on the television, guaranteed that study is paid for by the industry pushing the product, and the airtime to reveal the "good news" of the study is also paid.

Digging through the cracks in the research field is where you find interesting nuggets of truth. In a study on soy diets, they might find that adding walnuts to the diet had a surprising effect. This kind of research gets put out by people with keen eyes or sturdy hearts who are willing to dig through studies about other things.

The problem here is that the big money has an interest in making bigger money. Take Monsanto, for example. They're going to hire an army of researchers every year to develop positive studies about their pesticides and foods. They will pay big money to develop more genetically modified foods and extend their reach by patenting genetically modified foodstuffs, including animals. Nothing wrong with that; it's business. They will then own sole rights the world over to food. See, you can't patent food, but you can patent a genetic modification.

So many of the Big Companies have big money interests in making sure their big investments go through. That's where the lobbyists come in handy in Washington DC. They bribe our congressmen to pass legislation making their goals legal and punishing (usually through excessive taxation) small companies with bright and healthy approaches.

But what does this mean to food? Simple fact is, nearly all studies are a fabrication that come to a predetermined conclusion. If a Big Company wants you to eat more of their food that is loaded with addictive substances, they will commission a study saying "find us results that show there is no harmful side effects to eating our product."

See where this goes? The scientist on the other end needs to come to that conclusion or he's out of a job. He will do his best to justify the funding, finding anything he can to get to that conclusion – legitimately, of course.

This leads into the **detrimental studies**. **"Eggs are bad."** *No, they're not*, but we all remember the studies. Question is, who won? Who lost? A whole ton of small, independent farmers went out of business and were snapped up by the Big Corporations who are now happily selling those same eggs with "new studies" showing eggs are actually good after all. Remember all the farm closures in the 1980s? Who profited? And were those studies designed to pinch the small farmer so that they were foreclosed and/or forced to sell? Now almost all eggs are factory-style horror stories you wouldn't want to feed to a dog.

Many, many studies use *correlation* rather than *causation* for their conclusions. The egg study was that eggs were bad because of cholesterol and fat – and they left out all the pertinent truth of the matter and the study made eggs look bad.

Here's a little story to illustrate what I mean about correlation instead of causality. Here's my study: 55% of people who breathe die of heart attacks. Thus, if you cease breathing you can cut your heart attack risk by..." Get it? That's correlation and it means nothing. It means absolutely nothing. Next time you hear about a new study involving risk of death, pay close attention; you'll see these studies in a new light.

Here's another example of correlation, if on the funny side:

Vodka and ice will ruin your kidneys.
Rum and ice will ruin your liver.
Whiskey and ice will ruin your heart.
Gin and ice will ruin your brain.
Coke and ice will ruin your teeth.

That dang ice is lethal! Warn all your friends: Lay off the ice!

That is correlation. Most studies you see on television are hyped-up correlation.

The egg study left out the fact that eggs are high in High Density Lipoprotein, which actually keeps the heart healthy, your arteries smooth and pliable and everything functioning normally[9]. High in fat? Sure. Eggs are a great source of Omega 3 Fatty Acids, which are essential to good health[10]. I will have more to say on the Omega Fatty Acids in the next chapter.

EGGS:

• High in Omega 3 Fatty Acids – good for heart and arteries.
• A source of Vitamin D – essential for your immune system and can alleviate chronic back pain. Helps keep bones and teeth strong.
• High in Vitamin B2, B6, B7,and B12. Vitamin B's promote healthy heart, liver, eyes, skin. They help you metabolize fat and protein.

•	A source of Vitamin A – fights infections and is a wonderful antioxidant. Good for the eyes.
•	Excellent and primary source of lutein – prevents macular degeneration and cataracts.
•	Good source of choline – good for your brain, cardiovascular system and nervous system.
•	A source of sulphur – grows your hair, stronger nails.

There is no legitimate limit to egg intake. "Studies" suggest three per week. Ridiculous. A 3-egg omelet every day for breakfast is a great way to eat in the morning. I eat a 2-egg scramble every morning. I sauté some mushrooms and either fresh spinach or broccoli in olive oil. I scramble the egg into that and place it over a big slice of raw red onion. I'll describe why those particular foods in a different chapter.

Eggs are best eaten cooked. The reason is that there is a chemical (*avidin*) in the white that blocks your body from absorbing the Biotin (B7) in the egg yolk. Cooking (scrambling, frying or hard-boiling) neutralizes the avidin and allows your body to absorb this very crucial B Vitamin. Raw egg whites are just a bad idea as they will go through your system leeching out any Biotin you have ingested. Biotin deficiency can result in hair loss, seizures, lack of muscle coordination and lack of muscle tone, muscle cramps and pain.

CNN, CBS, FOX all ran blazing headlines in 2012 that a single egg was as bad as smoking a cigarette – building arterial plaque[11]. *Horse poop.* The "study" is correlation. What we have to ask is what kind of eggs? Factory cage eggs? What else did they eat with that egg yolk? Toast? Hash browns? What did they eat for lunch? Dinner? None of these questions were addressed.

Allow me to finish this particular chapter with this: somebody wants you **un**healthy. There is **huge** money in the medical industry – billions and billions in just one pill each year. Those who are on prescriptions were on the following eye-popping intake in 2006: 12 to 17 prescription drugs[12]. The profits are staggering. Back in the early 1990s, I was watching Newt Gingrich on a financial show and he said that the future of money was healthcare[13]. Would a huge medical conglomerate commission a study to keep you from eating healthier so you live long, unhealthy lives while they siphon off your wealth through "medications" no one ever needed before?

Think about that.

Next chapter will further clear up the horse-poop flung around by these studies lumping all fats together as bad.

CHAPTER 3

In the previous chapters we know this:

- Wheat – very bad. Don't eat, don't touch, don't even have memories of it
- Eggs – very good for you – but I am not done talking about eggs!
- Newt Gingrich: "The future of money is health care."

That's right, I'm not done with eggs.

In this chapter I want to introduce the subject that most of us probably know a lot about: fats. In particular the **Essential Fatty Acids**. I will also talk about **meat**. And **eggs** again. I will try to be brief, as I am sure knowledgeable readers have heard all this before.

What most of us know is that Omega 3 fatty acids are good. The body most efficiently uses Omega 3s to convert the ALA to EPA and also into DHA[14]. Omega 3s have been shown to reduce inflammation, shrink tumors, reduce obesity, eliminate brain disorders[15].

Most of us also understand that too much Omega 6 Fatty Acids are not too good. Omega 6s can cause inflammation, cause cardiovascular diseases, cause mental disorders and cause cancer[16].

We would do better to aim for foods high in Omega 3s and very low in Omega 6s. But there's a problem. Fish, red meat and eggs are sources of Omega 3s. So here is the egg thing again and the problem with eating eggs. Yes, I know, I said eggs are good. Hang on a sec.

Most huge farm conglomerates factory-process their production. We've all heard the horror stories of caged chickens living their lives doing nothing but producing eggs inside a tiny cage. They can't move, can't walk, nothing. They are fed a special diet of grains. Like corn. Well, guess what? Corn is high in Omega 6s and almost all corn is now genetically modified. Not only does corn thus contribute to inflammation, cancers, and obesity, but the Omega 6s are passed along into whatever eats it. Short version: factory eggs are higher in Omega 6s than 3s[17].

Avoid all the major brands of eggs. Luckily for me, nearly all eggs produced in Montana come from the Mennonites (like the Amish, but they drive cars).

Here's a short and ugly introduction to a term we all trust: **organic**. Why ugly? Well, the USDA has certain rules for the "organic" label and it isn't for our health benefit but specifically to make the food more costly. You see, it is cheaper to grow an organic tomato. So why does it cost almost twice as much in the grocery store? Organic growers must certify their products are organic, through third party means, and pay for that "organic" stamp on their label. The government has made sure the hoops to jump through are numerous enough to make a cheaper and better food cost more. The higher the cost, the more likely you'll grab the chemically fertilized version that costs more to grow.

Organic eggs: chickens can't be treated with hormones or antibiotics. Their feed must be non-genetically modified and grown organically. Sounds good, right? Mostly. Organic does not mean free range and organic does not necessarily mean that the chicken farmer can't use a feed high in Omega 6s.

Free Range eggs: these chickens are allowed to roam and eat whatever they want, including feed. The farmer does not need to abide by any other rule. He can inject them with hormones, antibiotics and whatever else the big factories do.

Cage-Free eggs: means nothing really. It's a salve to the conscience of the buyer. Running around on a concrete floor in a crammed-full barn is considered "cage free." That's it.

What we want, ideally, and good luck finding them (although they are out there), are **organic, free-range eggs**. If you can find both claims on the egg carton, you have found your egg.

This leads to meat, and in particular beef. Regular grocery-store beef is a no-no. Think of the factory again. The hormones and antibiotics in the beef (rBGH/BST) are manufactured by MONSANTO[18]. Yep. All genetically modified for your health... or, is it **their profits**? Bovine growth hormone has been shown to cause breast cancer, colon cancer, and prostate cancer and Monsanto knew all about it during development[19]. That means your typical jug of milk, your beef, your hamburger, your cheese and even butter should be avoided entirely. Not only for rBGH, but also that the cows are fed an extremely unhealthy diet of genetically modified grains – meaning, the cows are high in Omega 6s, and so is their milk, beef, cheese, and butters.

But there are alternatives.

Harder to find are cows raised without the hormones and antibiotics. Here is something of which to be aware: "**natural beef**" means minimally processed. That's all. It can be treated with Monsanto's rBGH hormone. "**Organic beef**" is what you want to find (no added hormones), although here is where "organic" can fail: organic cows must be fed organic feed, which could include grains high in Omega 6s.

So what you want to find is **organic grass-fed beef**. This type of meat is high in Omega 3s.

Here is another ugly little secret. Your restaurants, primarily supplied through a few major restaurant food supply corporations are going to deliver to you typical hormone-treated meat. It takes a conscientious owner/manager to supply and unfortunately charge more for real grass-fed steaks. I simply can't find anything to eat at restaurants anymore.

Further along the Omega 3 and Omega 6 chain are the fats we use as oils. The short version: extra virgin olive oil, avocado oil and organic raw coconut oil are the only oils you should ever use, ever, period, no exceptions. Here's why none of the others: corn oil, canola oil, soybean oil, palm oil, whatever are all packed high in Omega 6s. Further and just as important, cooking with those oils causes those oils to become trans-fats (they are partially hydrogenated to begin with for thickness)[20]. Trans fats clog your arteries, cause obesity, cause cancer and cause unsightly mustaches on women. Yes, that last was a joke. Trans-fats: very bad.

A couple of points:

The FDA allows packages to claim "no trans fats" or "Zero Trans Fats" when the food inside does indeed contain trans fats. Why? The FDA allows food manufacturers to claim a pre-cooked state for the oil or trans-fats at a low measure per serving[21]. Read your labels. Soybean oil used in preparation **is** a trans-fat. All the time, every single time, without exception.

Canola oil comes from the genetically modified rapeseed plant – a highly toxic plant to humans[22]. And don't be fooled by the label "organic" on anything having to do with canola[23].

Olive, avocado and coconut oil have higher heat tolerances before becoming trans-fats. You can deep-fry in coconut, so most of your cooking temperatures should be very safe. More on that in another chapter.

Maybe I should finish this chapter with why GM (genetically modified) foods are bad. Most might already know this. But here is a totally laymen's-term synopsis. Our bodies absorb information from what we eat into our RNA (think of it like our body's ink) which then transfers changes to our DNA (think of it like our body's paper). We are what we eat? But it is true. God made plants and animals a certain way and our digestive tracts to process those things a certain way. A genetically modified food is not well-accepted by the body. In fact, GM food causes severe gut cramps in me. In fact, anything that causes gut cramps should be your warning signal that your body cannot absorb the nutrients and digest it like it should. Anyhow, GM foods have been firmly implicated in all kinds of cancers, Alzheimer's, diabetes, and more. Is that why there is such an enormous explosion in these maladies? We're wrecking our own DNA eating GM foods and wrecking our health.

Your typical restaurant is going to be serving whatever is cheapest to get. GM foods will be on the menu. Bread? GM wheat (ALL wheat is GM). Cooking oil? Canola (GM) or corn (GM). Cheeseburger? The bread is GM, the cheese treated with rBGH, the meat treated with the hormone and cooked in the GM trans-fat oil. The ketchup full of corn syrup (GM), the mustard filled with MSG (more on that later), the lettuce from China and filled with fecal bacteria (human poop), and the tomato possibly GM. There is a push to get all tomatoes GM by Monsanto, of course.

Depressing huh? As I said earlier, I just cannot find anything to eat in a restaurant anymore. Next chapter I will continue on with meats and fish.

CHAPTER 4

Just to recap:

- Wheat – very bad. Don't eat, don't touch, don't even have memories of it
- Eggs – very good for you – but I am still not done talking about eggs!
- Grass-fed organic beef is great! Regular beef is very bad
- Coconut, avocado, and olive oils are the only oils you should use for cooking
- Newt Gingrich: "The future of money is health care."

So in this one I will continue a little bit with **meat** and will also talk about the **dairy**. Throwing **coffee** in this one, too, earlier than I had planned, but eggs and coffee should go together, right?

Continuing with meat, let's look beyond beef meat. Here is where we suffer a little less, with some precaution. Pork is generally decent. By law, pigs cannot be treated with growth hormones[24]. I'm sure

Big Money Pharaceuticals are busy bribing congress to overturn that with the push behind Somatotropin, the porcine growth hormone[25]. Monsanto already tried to patent the pig – no, that is not a joke. The patent was a little more specific than that – attempting to secure the rights to a genetic marker in pigs directly related to growth[26]. Which is scary to me because that means someone, somewhere has already GM'd a pig and who knows how soon before it enters our food chain. There are plenty of news stories available about GM pigs. Thankfully, hopefully, they are not yet in our foodchain.

But so far, pork is good. No hormones, no antibiotics (unless they get sick), no GM (yet). It might be safer to get your pork from a smaller brand name or small farmer. This is where you can find a local butcher and ask him about local pigs and grass-fed beef; he'll know exactly what you're talking about.

Just to illustrate the silly pricing, one pound of grass-fed beef at Safeway is $7.00. Preposterous. Safeway regular beef (Select) is all factory – full of hormones and antibiotics. Blech. Stuff stinks, too, for $3.47/lb. At a smaller store, I can find grass-fed beef for $4.37/lb. Only a dollar more expensive. Easily affordable, especially when you consider you won't be paying the doctors tens of thousands of dollars to ignore what's wrong with you and prescribe pills. Prescriptions are far more expensive than grass-fed beef and they don't taste good, either. Shop around or find a butcher.

Pork is often sold as sausage, hot dogs, salami, ham and bacon. Each of these has different considerations.

Pork sausage: if you can find pure pork with maybe some salt or pepper, good. Once they add in dextrose, "spices" or "natural flavorings" (I will talk more about those later), drop the package. Let someone else pick it up.

Pork hot dogs: forget it. They all have dextrose. Dextrose in food is pure GM[27]. They also all have other chemicals you don't want. You can, however, find "Open Nature" Uncured Beef hot dogs and those have no bad ingredients at all.

Salami: forget it. They all have dextrose. That means pepperoni, too.

Ham: This is a good food choice, with a couple considerations. Most hams are cured with "flavorings" (bad), commercial salt (bad), caramel coloring (very bad), sodium nitrite/nitrate (could be bad, depends), and maybe sugar (very bad). More on those substances later. For the ham to be good, simply slice off the outer layer. Cut it off, throw it away and don't even feed it to your poor dog. Ham is a good source of B Vitamins. Don't go for "honey-baked" or any of that nonsense. You don't need the fructose corn syrups in it.

Bacon: this is a good food choice, despite all the negatives you hear. Bacon does not make you fat. Nuh uh, never. But there is a danger.

DANGER: Bacon has been said to cause cancer. No, it doesn't. If you read farther into whatever study done, you will find mention of the nitrates and nitrites used in curing the pork. There is nothing wrong with sodium nitrate or sodium nitrite. In fact, celery is loaded with sodium nitrite in its natural state. The problem with nitrites and nitrates causing cancer is not ingesting them, **but how you cook them**. At high temperatures sodium nitrite and nitrate transform into nitrosamines, a very cancerous substance. It's the nitrosamines that cause cancer, not the nitrites or nitrates. So, do not char your food. Do not go for the crispy bacon by cooking it on high or even medium. I set my bacon in a small blob of olive oil and turn the pan on low. The bacon almost bakes. It takes about two hours to cook the bacon to an even crispness – not charred crisp – and it is a nice golden brown color. Start your bacon early. Then use the bacon grease to cook your egg and throw some fresh spinach into that grease as well. Note: you do not have to suffer a two hour bacon-cook time – it was just an example. But do not cook your bacon on anything other than the upper end of **low** temperature. You can get nice bacon in about twenty minutes.

Animal fat is very good for you and does not make you fat! Really. The body uses fats to properly digest food and metabolize fat and proteins in your body to keep you trim and lean[28].

Uh oh, getting off the beaten path here, but I have to. Eating fat does not make you fat. But let me recap a very short version of the misunderstood Atkins Diet, okay? In case any of you missed it. Whatever we eat gets broken down and absorbed into the blood stream not as fat, but SUGAR. Glucose, to be exact. Our body uses that for energy. If not used in a few hours, it gets turned into glycogen and stored temporarily for burning when we're out of glucose. Twenty-four hours after it becomes glycogen, if not

used, it will be stored in your adipose tissues as fat[29].
Sugar (excess blood sugar) makes you fat. Fat does not.

I remember some ditzy gal who came into my game store when I had it and she was pushing athletic memberships at her place. She put three quarters into my candy machine and took a bunch of Red Hots. "Oooh! I love these," she said. "You can eat them all day long because there's no fat!" This was a fitness instructor who went to college and got a degree... Pardon me while I roll my eyes.

Here is an interesting related story. Olive oil is a fat, and considered "fattening" to the food pyramid crowd. Coconut oil even moreso. Things used to be deep fried in coconut oil. Potato chips forty years ago? Did they make you fat? Nope. But anyway, a couple of bright egghead labcoats got it in their food-pyramid-fat-makes-you-fat brains (brains?) and set about feeding a whole bunch of coconut oil to some pigs that they would sell as super-fat monstrosities and they would make millions. Guess what? The fattest of all "fattening" oils, coconut oil, produced an entire herd of lean pigs[30]. That's right. The idiots had to give up and go back to corn-feed. Our bodies process fat better for energy than carbs or sugars.

Anyway. On with meats.

Fish: freshwater fish *only* and never any kind of fish from China. Ocean fish with Fukushima radiation floating all over the world (as far as the Mediterranean now) is just asking for a heavy dose of Cesium. That kind of radioactive isotope is absorbed directly into your bones, providing you a lifetime of glowing green and all the ill health effects of radiation poisoning. **Tuna**? Forget it. **Salmon**? I love salmon. Forget it. Anything from the ocean – **shrimp, clams**... forget it. Some people claim the Fukishima radiation exposure from tuna is less than that of a banana, but these are extrapolations of exposure levels of only one thousand times the safe limit. For example, the highly publicized study that proclaimed "Tuna is Safe" supposes only **4 Bq** of Cesium per kilogram. The inconvenient truth is that the Bq levels of Cs are now over **40,000,000** in kelp beds and working up the food chain[31]. That's right, the media and government are hyping that it's perfectly safe to eat all kinds of seafood while ignoring the fact that radiation levels are over *ten million times worse than they are admitting*. And Fukushima is still pumping hush-hush horrific amounts of radiation into the ocean. This is an apocalypse of Biblical proportions. Never again eat seafood. I cannot stress this enough.

Conversely, sea salt actually helps clean radiation from the body (sea salt does not absorb cesium or any other radioactive particle in the first place)[32].

Fish from China are always horribly polluted[33] because they are raised in very unclean farms and fed a diet of chicken poop and human poop[34]. Check your labels for country of origin.

Chicken: an excellent food. However, do not ever buy the big name brand chicken and not frozen chicken, either. The "big name" farms add arsenic to their chicken to give it a nice color. The frozen chicken has a glaze that is loaded with MSG, arsenic, and other stuff you wouldn't even give Osama bin

Laden as food. Buy chicken that claims no hormones or antibiotics. Buy it fresh in the package. Some brands will brag about free-range chicken content. You want those, not the big names.

Other meat. Buffalo is excellent and so is venison if they slaughtered it right (no gamey taste). Neither of those can be raised like factory cows. Buffalo has a wonderful deep-beef flavor that is as close to a good clean beef taste as I've found. Unfortunately, buffalo is expensive at around $6 per pound that I don't buy it anymore. Turkey sure tastes good, but the modern turkey has been crossbred into the big breasted bird we see today and unfortunately gets sick easy. Turkey is fed a steady stream of antibiotics and unhealthy drugs to cause them to produce more meat[35].

Dairy – in particular milk, butter and cheese.

Milk: I avoid it, but if you really want milk, buy organic whole milk, and raw unpasteurized if you can get it. Here's why: organic milk comes from organically-raised cows and has a decent amount of Omega 3 fatty acids. Further, the nutrients are in the fat. When you buy non-fat pastuerized milk, you're not only wasting your health-money, but ingesting more of the water that contains pesticides, herbicides and all the other crap that poisons our water. Pasteurization was good for its time, but is a poor practice in modern times. The heating kills the nutrients in the milk making it fairly worthless. The reason I avoid milk is that we don't need it and it isn't natural for one species to require or need the milk of another. You don't see dogs chasing down pregnant

30

rats trying to get their milk. So, organic whole milk, preferably raw.

Butter: I love butter. I'll cook with it, slather it on veggies. Butter is an excellent fat to eat with foods. But, look for butter that boasts on the package that it comes from cows not treated with rBGH. Challenge, Kirkland, and Tillamook butters come to mind. I'm talking real butter not margarine. Margarine is made from petroleum. Never, ever eat margarine.

Cheese: Almost all cheese is treated with annatto for coloring. Pick up a block of "pure" cheddar cheese and see what I mean. Avoid, avoid, avoid. Annatto is another name for MSG (more on MSG later). Avoid all big-name cheese as it will be coming from cows treated with rBGH. I was fortunate to find a cheese by "Open Nature" that contains none of the MSG or other harmful preservatives and comes from cows not treated with all the crap. Tillamook white cheese also is a good non-rBGH cheese. Sliced sandwich-ready cheese in convenient little plastic wraps? You must be kidding. Forget it. I'll have more to say on plastic later.

Let's wrap this chapter up with coffee and cocoa. Yep, cocoa.

Coffee: If it has a bunch of "appa" and "cino" names, forget it. That is the perfect way to ruin something good while spending more money consuming it. Also, the famous neurosurgeon Dr. Blaylock warned that some of those high-end pricey coffees come from coffee beans soaked in horse urine. Avoid the pricey coffee. But coffee is a wonderful beverage if done right and consumed in quantities that are sparing. Here's the dirt on coffee. Best drank black. Don't ruin it with sugars or sweeteners. Everybody has heard that blueberries have the highest antioxidant of any food? Not true. Then it was cranberries. Not true. Coffee has something like 14 times the antioxidant content in a single cup compared to a cup of blueberries – and who eats a whole cup of blueberries? Coffee, caffeinated, is a wonderful pick-me-up in the morning packed with antioxidants[36]. It was even supposed that coffee won the Civil War for the Union forces because they drank it every morning while the South couldn't get any through the blockade. Ha. Coffee also stimulates peristalsis, the movement in your bowels to make you go sit on the toilet. In other words, it can help relieve constipation. More on constipation later! **But, there is a danger to coffee**. Coffee is a diuretic, meaning that it can leech the water out of your system. This can lead to swelling and inflammation and also constipation and other issues you don't want and that a doctor would love to give you a pill for. Two to four cups a day is not bad, but I would not go beyond that and certainly make sure you get adequate water intake later.

Further, do not drink your coffee with your meals! You want to be taking vitamins with your meals and coffee (the caffeine in coffee) inhibits or blocks the absorption (or causes depletion) of the following nutrients: Vitamin D; iron; B-vitamins (except it actually aids in absorbing B-12); manganese; zinc; copper; potassium; and magnesium. Caffeine also inhibits the activity of Vitamin A. For those who pop their vitamin packs with those caffeinated "energy drinks," they're wasting their time.

I make my coffee with cocoa. I buy organic coffee beans and grind them myself. The fact that I bought an organic bag of them made me wonder if other coffee was treated with something unhealthy – turns out I was right[37]. I used to love Folgers but it now comes in a plastic tub. More on plastic later! Mixed into the coffee beans for grinding, I put a half teaspoon of pure cocoa powder. I'm not talking something sweet. This is baking powder, totally unsweetened. Not Hersheys. Not Nestles (Nestles owns Hersheys) Not Mars or any other big-name chocolatier[38]. They were bragging about how their cocoa was going to be grown genetically modified starting this year. Bragging. However, chocolatiers were already using genetically modified sugar beets for their sugar. In fact, anything with "sugar" on the label should be completely avoided as it will be from genetically modified sources.[39] I use organic baking cocoa powder. Cocoa is something like 7 times higher in antioxidants than blueberries. But don't go out and buy processed chocolate. No no no no no. "But a candy bar tastes good." Maybe for someone still addicted to the chemicals. The stuff tastes like axle grease to me now.

The next chapter will be about **estrogen** and **vegetables**.

CHAPTER 5

A short recap:

• Wheat – very bad. Don't eat, don't touch, don't even have memories of it
• Eggs – very good for you – but I am not done talking about eggs!
• Grass-fed organic beef is great! Regular beef is very bad
• Coconut, avocado, and olive oils are the only oils you should use for cooking.
• Don't char your meat
• Coffee is good for you, sparingly
• Avoid all ocean seafood
• Newt Gingrich: "The future of money is health care."

This chapter is going to be primarily about **estrogen**, the female hormone (but also male). I will also be mentioning **plastics** in relation to them and also **vegetables**.

Don't get bored yet, this is one of the most crucial aspects to grasp about obesity, ill-health, and the desire to ram your car into the slow-poke ahead of you. Yes, seriously, and I'll explain why.

Sure, processed sugar is totally evil and does nothing but sweeten your food with dead, un-nutritional calories. But estrogen plays a huge role alongside sugar. Most know estrogen as a womanly thing, but not only is it something in men, but also in a balance with other hormones, though at different levels between the sexes. Women used to operate on a balance of progesterone, estrogen and testosterone. But nowadays, we're coming out of the womb already seriously out of whack. Men also have estrogen, but should be having more testosterone. Estrogen imbalance (too much) in men causes man-boobs, a pear-shaped body, impotence and one medical source I read suggested a shrinking male part.

In women, too much estrogen is causing an increased risk of miscarriages, increased PMS symptoms, depression, thyroid dysfunction, fibrocystic breasts, weight gain and irregular menstrual cycles. That's right, weight gain[40].

Eat like a bird? Gain five pounds? Look at a cookie and gain five more? *Think* about a cookie and gain another five? Your culprit then isn't overeating but your estrogen – and that goes for men, too. Our metabolisms do slow down with age, but some women I've known can't even eat a single cracker per day without adding more fat.

I need to take a short detour back to calories. Calories are totally worthless. Any Masters Degree Health Graduate can tell you I'm wrong. But I'm not and here's why: a calorie is a measurement of energy produced. That's all. It has no other relation. But I tell you that a calorie of soy and a calorie of beef have totally different effects on the body. One will make me fat, the other will make me skinny. If I ate 1000 calories of soybeans per day I would gain fat no matter how much I exercised – not to mention that soy is the culprit in bodily inflammation: a condition extremely unhealthy. If I ate a 1000 calories of butter per day, I could lay around and watch the fat melt away. Forget energy – food has different effects, thus calories are worthless.

Before you scratch your chin, consider this. Certain types of foods increase your estrogen levels. Others decrease them.

Here's what excess levels of estrogen do in men and women: estrogen will cause your body to store fat by making what I call "estrogenic tissues" - or fat tissues that store your estrogen. Sure, sounds bad, but it's worse, far worse, than that. Estrogenic tissues force your body to make even more estrogenic tissues even if you don't eat any more "calories." More and more and more. Once you begin building those tissues, forcing more to be built, and more, it is very hard to stop them. Also, these tissues are storing all the toxins you eat in your food. This is why you can't look at a cookie and not gain five pounds. Guess what? You don't even need to look at the cookie to gain five pounds because your body is doing it for you anyway, converting anything you eat or drink into more estrogenic tissues. It is an avalanche-snowball effect that grows and grows without stopping[41].

Starving yourself is not the answer, though you do limit the amount of fat you gain. Starvation diets are the stupidest ways to lose weight. The body goes further out of balance being robbed of nutrients you need to even begin shedding that fat.

The key here is to eat foods that don't add to your estrogen and in women to eat foods that add to your progesterone. In men, eat foods that help in testosterone production.

High estrogen foods to avoid:

- **All soy**. Extremely estrogenic
- Sunflower seeds
- Alfalfa sprouts. Extremely estrogenic
- Beer

Many women getting along in years take herbs to alleviate peri-menopause, menopause, or post menopause problems. But it is so wrong what we have been told. Sure, the herbs are an effective salve to the emotions, wild mood swings and everything else. But guess what? They're making things worse and making you fatter. Nearly all of the common "health" herbs for women are highly estrogenic. Makes you feel good for a day, then makes you fatter. Remember, we want to decrease estrogen and increase progesterone in women. Herbs to avoid:

- blue cohosh
- black cohosh
- dong quai
- hops (beer again)
- lavender

- licorice
- motherwort leaf
- rhodiola rose root
- red clover blossom
- saw palmetto
- tea tree oil

Don't even use them in lotions. Ugh, lotions is another subject.

There are a few veggies you can eat that kill estrogenic tissues – forcing your body to burn them and shut them down permanently. Yep, **kill** them. The veggies would be **Brussels sprouts, broccoli, cauliflower, kale, cabbage and turnips**. They contain a nutrient called indole-3-carbinol and it is your primary estrogen fighter in food[42].

There are no foods that directly supply women with progesterone, but you can eat certain foods that help your body build more and thus bring you back into balance.

You want to eat more of these:

- Foods high in B6: Eggs; ham; beef; walnuts; bananas; spinach; beans; and potatoes
- Vitamin C – but forget a pill supplement. *They're worthless.* More on that later.
- Foods high in Zinc: Beef; liver; and dark chocolate (unsweetened).

Remember that the B Vitamins can cure depression[43]. B Vitamins can soothe all those anger issues...

About chocolate, don't go out and buy a candy bar. Just stop thinking about them. The cocoa has been so processed and killed with GM sugars that even sniffing one probably damages your health. Think I'm kidding? Anyhow, buy bakers chocolate, dark, unsweetened. Yeah, it's bitter at first. My wife and I have been eating a square a day for months now. Took about a week to develop a taste for it and after a few weeks they actually tasted good. Don't buy Hershey's or Nestles baking cocoa. Remember, they're genetically modified.

Personal anecdotal evidence: by following these simple steps my wife has been able to stop taking all those engineered for moody-women herbs. She eats chocolate, eats the same amount of food every day. She eats the foods I mentioned, but won't touch liver. Her mood swings are gone. Her irritability gone. She had started thickening up in the arms and thighs – typical of what most women think is "normal." She had also started swelling in her ankles and calves. The swelling is gone. The thickened areas are shrinking. All without exercise.

Once we remove things from our diet that cause us to be fat or bloated, our bodies will begin to restore a state of healthiness.

PROBLEM: exercise will make you feel really, really bad. There is a danger there, too. Strenuous exercise will release all those toxins (excitotoxins) from your fatty tissues and you'll get headaches, nausea, diarrhea maybe, constipation maybe, and could lead to maladies like cancer. Yep. I'm not saying exercise is bad. Strenuous exercise is bad. Walking is fine. No more than that. Swimming is good. If you feel you must exercise, keep it very, very light.

I said I would mention plastics and it has a very severe effect, but this chapter is already long. So plastics in the next one and I'll also talk about microwaves.

Your body is not your enemy; **you** are your own worst enemy by what you eat.

CHAPTER 6

A short recap:

- Wheat – very bad. Don't eat, don't touch, don't even have memories of it
- Eggs – very good for you
- Grass-fed organic beef is great! Regular beef is very bad
- Coconut, avocado, and olive oils are the only oils you should use for cooking
- Don't char your meat
- Coffee is good for you, sparingly
- Avoid all ocean seafood.
- Eliminate as many estrogens from your food as possible
- Eat lots of broccoli - not done talking about broccoli, either
- Newt Gingrich: "The future of money is health care."

This chapter is going to be a continuation of estrogen as I introduce **plastics**. Also going to talk about the **microwave**. Sometime I will have to get back to veggies – maybe next chapter.

Plastics have to be one of the most vile evils on the face of the planet. I have a chemist friend who is a chemist (PhD) in Pittsburgh. He tells me that chemists cannot use plastic in certain experiments because the plastic contaminates whatever products they are testing. Immediate contamination[44]. Plastic, even when new, constantly leech toxic chemicals into their surroundings[45]. Landfills continuously leak vinyl chloride, benzene, dioxins, phthalates, bisphenol-A, and formaldehyde. All of these are extremely toxic to humans.

Did you know all of these compounds are found in humans tested (phthalates and other toxins)? Not naturally – I'm talking accumulated over the years by exposure. If my chemist friend is correct, even the newest plastic is constantly emitting these chemicals.

What do these chemicals cause? Blech, so much you really don't want to know, but here's a short list:

- cancer, of course
- endometriosis
- neurological damage
- endocrine disruption
- birth defects and child developmental disorders
- reproductive damage
- immune system damage

- asthma
- multiple organ damage and failure

Those chemicals are also in flame retardants. Our poor young, we swaddle them in flame retardant blankets, diaper them in plastic, shove a vinyl (plastic) pacifier in their mouths, feed them from plastic bottles, give them plastic toys to play with. But I'll tell you something even more horrifying to comprehend a little later.

I wanted to introduce plastic not just because I hate plastic; it has a profound effect on our health because the plastic is extremely **estrogenic**[46]. And I mean extremely. **Dare I say right now**, your Tupperware alone, leeching all those estrogenic chemicals into your food is making you fat and you're not even eating it! "Hey look, how cute, I can burp the bowl." Gain a pound.

Almost every foodstuff is now packaged in plastic. Remember when bacon came in a box? Remember when meat came wrapped in heavy paper? Remember when Wheaties were just in a cardboard box and not in a plastic bag in the box? Guess what my wife and I saw last month: a cereal box wrapped in plastic. That's right, not only is the cereal inside packaged in plastic, but the cardboard outer box was then additionally wrapped in plastic. Ugh.

"Well," you say, "plastic keeps things fresh." It does, it does. Fresher longer, sure. But at what cost? The steady accumulation of toxic estrogens in your body?

Here's my recommendation.

Get rid of all your plastic containers, bowls, drinking cups – everything you use. Buy tin. Buy steel. Buy ceramics. Buy glass. I tear open all my plastic and dump whatever into glass. Or old coffee cans (though the lids are still plastic). Old glass peanut butter jars are wonderful. Make sure any container of whatever material does not come from China. I don't hate China, but they constantly send irradiated metal products, use toxic substances in almost everything they make, and just don't care[47].

I rip open all my meat and wrap it in freezer paper. Be careful! A very popular brand of freezer paper is plastic-coated. I tear open all my cheese and wrap it in wax paper. There is a good supply of wax-paper products at bigger stores.

Just let me repeat so it gets past our "I really don't want to know this" defense mechanism. **Plastics are extremely estrogenic** and are constantly emitting estrogenic compounds directly into you – making you fatter and sicker.

By the way, the cancer-causing success of BPA (bisphenol-A) is so resounding that it is now in all printer ink for your enjoyment. Grab that receipt? Gain a pound. Follow a printed sentence with your finger? Gain two. It is enough to make one go on a rampage.

Okay, here's the bombshell I considered one day. I have no proof of this. I can point to no study being done, having been done, and I really doubt anyone will *ever* commission such a study. So you just have to use your brains to judge what I am saying here. **Nylon** and **polyester** are petroleum (plastic) products. That's right. There's no nylon tree or polyester shrub we harvest. These two clothing substances come from the exact same toxic processes as all the rest of the plastics. Just as estrogenic because they contain all the same compounds[48]. Put on your socks? Gain a pound. Think about it. The more estrogen you introduce to your body, the more fatty estrogenic tissues you accumulate – which force your body to build more estrogenic tissues, and more and more and more.

I buy and wear only wool and cotton. I am ambivalent about cotton. Cotton is now genetically modified. We certainly want to avoid and never ingest anything made with cottonseed oil. But it probably doesn't hurt to wear it as you aren't wearing the seeds. In fact, I'll venture to say wearing cotton is perfectly safe. Just don't eat it.

I threw away all my polyester and nylon clothing. Some can't be avoided, like the elastic band in the socks or underwear. But you can limit it. Remove as much of this estrogenic clothing as possible and reduce your exposure.

Okay, on to the wonderful, dandy **microwave** (invented by the nazis, by the way and aren't all things nazi supposed to be evil?).

The microwave uses radiation to cook your food. It uses gamma radiation and a typical zap of your food is equivalent to 30 million chest x-rays. Sound healthy yet? I don't want 30 million chest x-rays. However, your food does not come out radioactive. Don't worry, it doesn't glow and it won't make you glow. What it does come out as is radioimetic. The radiation has created radiolytic products in your food. In effect, you have changed the food into a mutation of what it had been[48].

These irradiated foods we plop down and eat after a zap cause a short list of delightful effects[49]:

- cancer
- premature death
- reproductive dysfunction (male impotence and erectile dysfunction included)
- chromosomal abnormalities (**human mutation**)
- liver damage

By using the microwave, your food becomes somewhat indigestible. But don't think that is good because that might cause you to lose weight. Not only indigestible, but nuking your food destroys the vitamins and Essential Fatty Acids in what you are eating. You might as well gnaw on a decomposed rat. Well, that would probably be more healthy for you than eating microwaved food. Shoot, just scoop some roadkill up off the street. So the mutated food not only has little or no nutritional value, but your intestines do not like it. Irritable Bowel Syndrome is often the result. And the colon cancers, how wonderful. IBS is constipation and the inability of your intestines to properly function – such as when you do eat a healthy food, they just simply will not absorb the nutrients like they should.

Who wants cancer? Eat from a microwave and you shout out to the world that you not only want it, but look forward to it. Simply put, the microwave turns your food carcinogenic[50].

Throw the microwave away. It has absolutely no value at all or any kind of utility. "But but but, I heat my water in it." Stop it. For the cost of a microwave, just buy a water cooler for bottled water with a heat faucet on it. You get instant scalding hot water without the radiation.

That beautiful, so useful microwave on your counter? Throw it. Throw it. Throw it. Give it a kick, too. And toss the tellyvision with it.

Back to food next chapter. **Veggies** and **organics** and the dangers of them.

CHAPTER 7

A short recap:

- Wheat – very bad. Don't eat, don't touch, don't even have memories of it
- Eggs – very good for you
- Grass-fed organic beef is great! Regular beef is very bad
- Coconut, avocado, and olive oils are the only oils you should use for cooking.
- Don't char your meat
- Coffee is good for you, sparingly
- Avoid all ocean seafood
- Eliminate as many estrogens from your food as possible
- Eat lots of broccoli - not done talking about broccoli, either
- Eliminate as much plastic as possible – plastic is estrogenic
- Never use a microwave

- Newt Gingrich: "The future of money is health care."

This one is about **veggies** and **organics** again. Remember, the trick to getting your body working for you rather than against you is to limit its exposure to these horrid influences.

One other thing hearkening back to last chapter's plastics, the non-stick plastic coatings on your pans is leeching these chemicals directly into your food. Doesn't matter if the coating peels, it is emitting these chemicals new out of the box. I suggest all stainless steel cookware but not made in China – they use contaminated and sometimes radioactive metals. Cast iron is okay for women but men really need to limit their exposure to cast iron cooking. The iron in older men accumulates in the liver and can cause cirrhosis – even if they never drink alcohol.

So, **veggies**. We have all heard "wash your vegetables." Washing is good – it removes the pesticides and herbicides from the surface of the food. It also removes dust and dirt that may be contaminated from Fukushima radiation. Washing removes the radioactive particles. But there are dangers. If you wash with unfiltered tap water, you're adding chemicals and the aluminum and the fluoride in the water bind to your veggies so that you ingest them directly. Unfiltered tap water also contains BPA, a whole host of prescription drugs reclaimed from people peeing them out into the sewage system[51].

Don't shake your head. All municipalities use treated sewage water to supplement the water supply.

A reverse osmosis filter removes all that garbage and your veggies will be clean.

Probably the most popular veggie is **lettuce**. A nice head of iceberg lettuce is probably the most popular purchase by people who believe they are health-conscious. You know what? Lettuce is probably the least nutritious vegetable there is. It's worthless. I wouldn't feed it to my pet rats.

Want a salad? Want that green on your breadless burger? Use raw **spinach** instead. Not only does it taste better, but spinach is packed with vital nutrients. One cup has all your Vitamin A and K for the day, is bursting with manganese and folate, and is a good source of magnesium. Magnesium can lower your blood pressure in as little as two hours. Spinach is also an excellent source of beta-carotene, a powerful antioxidant that improves cardiovascular health, guards against lung cancers and oral cavities, destroys prostate cancer, and reduces the risk of ovarian cancer in women.

Couple little tricks to spinach. Most of the vitamins are water soluble. If you boil your spinach, you're losing your vitamins. Eat it raw. But not just raw. The beta carotene is fat soluble – chewing it won't do you any good. To release the beta carotene in spinach, fry it lightly in your bacon grease, or a small pool of olive oil. Top your eggs with that and reap the benefits. So eat both raw and fat-cooked spinach.

Canned spinach is boiled and is really only useful for its vegetable fiber and I would question whether or not the vegetable was first sprayed with

Roundup (highly neuro-toxic) or washed with unfiltered tap water. I can't help but look at canned spinach with a sneer of suspicion and disgust.

So I am going to depart here from veggies while I am on spinach and talk about **constipation**. Spinach is a great source of fiber. If you are taking any kind of fiber supplements, stop immediately. Yes, you heard me – stop taking all fiber supplements immediately. The only thing that fiber is doing is creating extra-large stools that are themselves difficult to pass. Fiber also scrapes up the intestines and irritates the bowels. You get all the fiber you need from your veggies and fruits – believe me, plenty. Taking fiber supplements will cause IBS (Irritable Bowel Syndrome) or constipation and abdominal pain[52]. Throw the supplements away. "But I'm constipated! Fiber helps me go." No, it does not. All that fiber is doing is making a bigger stool and scraping the heck out of your intestines. **The absolute #1 cure for constipation is spinach.** Even the worst cases of constipation can be cured by eating spinach. Eat it every day. Another method to helping relieve constipation along with eating plenty of spinach is to raise your knees. Even lifting them by raising your feet on their tiptoes helps create a straighter passage for a stool. The typical toilet-seat level misaligns the rectal canal and can impede stool passage. Drink water – at least two or more big glasses per day along with all your other fluids. Your constipation will be a memory in a few months; your intestines take time to heal from all that fiber damage.

Further, fiber and teas that help you go and even suppositories create a dependence on them so that eventually you have to use them to even go. Stop the insanity. Stop creating a condition of constipation, unless you like being constipated. With spinach, raising the knees and drinking plenty of water, regularity can return in as little as three to four weeks. How does a bowel movement everyday sound? I know some people who go once every three weeks. End the torture and let your intestines heal now that you know the truth.

Back to foods.

Organics. Pound for pound, organic veggies and fruits are shown to have a higher nutritional content and none of the pesticides and herbicides so toxic to humans[53]. Your body will love you for eating them. But, wash wash wash. We still don't know what's being sprayed in those chemtrails and tests have shown toxic chemicals laying on everything after a chem-spray. I don't want to argue if chemtrails are real or not – especially when our own governments have admitted chemtrails are real[54]. Our officials may say they are for weather engineering, but why the deadly neuro-toxic chemicals? All I know is that several tests were done by labs on the droplets that accumulated after a so-called chemtrail. They were loaded with barium and aluminum.

Barium can cause heart arrhythmias, respiratory failure, gastrointestinal dysfunction, paralysis, muscle twitching, and elevated blood pressure. Barium also deactivates your body's immune response to things like H1N1[55]. Is there collusion between government and big money pharmaceuticals? Makes you wonder, doesn't it. I remember some state governments mandating everyone getting the swine flu shot a couple years ago and the federal government ordered 10s of millions of flu shots. The taxpayer footed the bill, of course, but there was no swine flu epidemic as promised, even though millions of Americans refused to get the shots. However, the pharmaceutical company had already pocketed its billions[56]. So make sure to wash even your organics.

Further, and it might sound odd, but wash your oranges before you peel them and here's why: all oranges are sprayed with Bonide (malathion) for shipment. Kills any bugs on them that might do dirty work on the fruit while it's moving from point A to point B. If you peel your orange, you've got whatever is on the outside on your hands, now touching the stuff you're putting in your mouth. Consider anything you need to peel or open as contaminated.

Other than lettuce, all veggies provide you benefits you can't get in a packaged meal. You'll find mushrooms in the veggie section. Buy them and eat them raw. Also saute them and throw them on your food. Mushrooms protect you against diseases and infections, as they are full of proteins, vitamins, minerals, amino acids, antibiotics and antioxidants. They lower your cholesterol, ward against breast and prostate cancers, fight diabetes and help you lose fat[57].

If you can't handle mushrooms, that's okay. My wife hates them too.

But if you have to snack and you like mushrooms, what better snack? Ditch the Doritos –

grocery store "snacks" are filled with ingredients designed to make you addicted and sick.

Here's another word on salads. If you decide to change your salad routine and use spinach instead, make sure you don't put any store-bought "dressing" on it. Dressing, no-no, bad. Read the labels. The dressings are loaded with soy (estrogenic, makes you fat), MSGs (makes you fat), and refined sugars (causes diabetes). Plus, many of the dressings are bottled in plastic for an extra dose of estrogenic compounds.

By the way, all store-bought mayonnaise is now made using soy oil. I love mayo – make it myself sometimes using olive oil. But do yourself a favor and throw away all your store-bought mayonnaise – it's killing you.

Next chapter I will continue with **Onions** and **Potatoes**, touching on **Vitamin C** and the **Glycemic Index**. Whew... that'll be a load.

CHAPTER 8

A short recap:

- Wheat – very bad. Don't eat, don't touch, don't even have memories of it
- Eggs – very good for you
- Grass-fed organic beef is great! Regular beef is very bad
- Coconut, avocado, and olive oils are the only oils you should use for cooking.
- Don't char your meat
- Coffee is good for you, sparingly
- Avoid all ocean seafood.
- Eliminate as many estrogens from your food as possible
- Eat lots of broccoli - not done talking about broccoli, either
- Eliminate as much plastic as possible – plastic is estrogenic
- Never use a microwave
- Buy organic, but not from china

- Eat spinach both raw and lightly fried in a fatty oil (bacon grease, olive, coconut oils)
- Newt Gingrich: "The future of money is health care."

In this chapter we're going to look at four different things and I will have to be somewhat light in how I approach them or just these four could take enormous chapters each all by themselves.

The **Glycemic Index** is a measure of how food impacts your blood sugar. Blood sugar (glucose) is 100 on the index and everything is measured by how fast whatever you eat is converted into glucose.

Here are the Glycemic index ratings on sugars[58].

- Table sugar 60
- Corn syrup 75
- Dextrose 100
- **Maltodextrin 150 - the SUPER Sugar!**

Those last two are in just about every packaged food you buy. I'll be talking about packaged foods later. Also, corn syrup, Dextrose and Maltodextrin are genetically modified sweeteners.

Here's where we talk about **potatoes**. Most people might know that potatoes are a good way to fatten someone up. When my son went into the Army, the recruiter mentioned his low weight. Told him to eat a ton of potatoes. For a long time, I was against potatoes with a conviction bordering on hysterical fanaticism. But, the potato is actually an excellent source of vitamins, minerals and nutrients. Their minerals include very good amounts of manganese, magnesium, potassium, and phosphorous, and moderate amounts of iron, copper, zinc, and calcium. In terms of vitamins, a single serving of potatoes contains great amounts of vitamin C, folate, vitamin B6, and niacin, as well as good amounts of pantothenic acid, thiamin, vitamin K, and riboflavin.

There's that very important B-6 again.

But here's the problem. People go in and grab a plastic bag (remember when potatoes came in rough potato sacks?) of Russet potatoes. Russet, russet, russet. Well, guess what? The glycemic index of potatoes goes as follows: Russets baked, around 100. Russets boiled around 110. Red potatoes baked, around 55. Red potatoes boiled around 75.

Don't buy Russets. Buy red potatoes. Don't boil them. Either bake them (which kills some of the nutrients), or fry them lightly in olive or coconut oil. Fried potatoes retain more nutrients. And never peel the potato. The nutrients aren't exactly in the skin, but are very close to the surface of the potato. If you peel the thing, you'll also be removing that subsurface where all the best nutrients are. Slice those suckers up and fry them on low heat. Takes about ten minutes per side. I sprinkle turmeric on mine and douse them with pepper – more on spices later.

Onions. Don't like them? You can skip this then. Onions are a very good source of vitamin C, B6, biotin, chromium, calcium and dietary fiber. In addition, they contain good amounts of folic acid and vitamin B1 and K.

There's that very important B-6 again.

Onions are also high in antioxidants and red onions are the best source of quercitin in anything available. Quercitin has been shown to thin the blood, lower cholesterol, raise good-type HDL cholesterol, ward off blood clots, fight asthma, chronic bronchitis, hay fever, diabetes, atherosclerosis and infections and is specifically linked to inhibiting human stomach cancer. But guess what? You won't find that in the white onion. Also the quercitin is near the surface, where the pigments color the onion. Peel off the papery skin, but when it starts looking shiny, leave that part.

Vitamin C. I brought potatoes and onions up because it is a subject very dear to me. When I was a hermit in the 80s, I developed **scurvy**. When I had self-diagnosed it, I was able to locate some wild rose bushes and eat the rose hips. The infection in a cut cleared up in just two days. But I had to then consume later in years vast amounts of vitamin C supplements just to maintain a very precarious health. Then I found out supplements were worthless for vitamin C. Why? Because Asorbic Acid is not vitamin C! The scientist who discovered what we call vitamin C today identified seven different interactive substances within the C-Complex. Asorbic Acid is nothing more than a wrapper. Imagine buying a carton of eggs and getting only the shells. You're not getting eggs. Likewise, the scientist who identified C (Dr. Albert Szent-Georgi) said that Asorbic Acid on its own could never cure scurvy – whereas a single onion or potato could[59]. Because they contain real Vitamin C. If not all 7 parts of the C-Complex are in evidence, you do not have a functioning Vitamin C.

Your doctor likely won't tell you this because many of them don't know. Why don't they? It is a failure of the medical industry.

Since learning about Asorbic Acid being totally worthless, I have taken to eating either an apple or an orange per day, and a healthy cut of raw, red onion for my scrambled eggs. All infections have ceased. I have not yet fallen sick to the flu or cold as happened every single year (kids in school bring it home).

Got Vitamin C supplements? Throw them away. Ascorbic acid, if you didn't know, is synthesized from corn syrup – as if you needed another reason to avoid it. It is detrimental to your health[60]. Who wants useless, genetically modified vitamins? Don't ever take Vitamin C again – get the real thing from your foods.

I kept this chapter marginally short. Ha.

Next chapter I will talk about **spices** and **hot sauces**.

CHAPTER 9

A short recap:

- Wheat – very bad. Don't eat, don't touch, don't even have memories of it
- Eggs – very good for you
- Grass-fed organic beef is great! Regular beef is very bad
- Coconut, avocado, and olive oils are the only oils you should use for cooking
- Don't char your meat
- Coffee is good for you, sparingly.
- Avoid all ocean seafood.
- Eliminate as many estrogens from your food as possible
- Eat lots of broccoli - not done talking about broccoli, either
- Eliminate as much plastic as possible – plastic is estrogenic
- Never use a microwave
- Buy organic, but not from china

- Eat spinach both raw and lightly fried in a fatty oil (bacon grease, olive, coconut oils)
- Eat red potatoes and red onions for the most nutrient value
- Newt Gingrich: "The future of money is health care."

This chapter is spices and hot sauces. Man loves to have certain spices in his dishes and the history of spice is as long as man himself. To buy spices, except for salt and pepper, don't waste your time buying it at the store. There are places online I find by doing a search for "buy spices online" and will sell to anyone even at wholesale pricing. Grocery stores will charge you twelve times as much for a tiny plastic jar of spice when you can get it by the pound or more.

I'm going to run through **salt** real quick. We all know and have heard we get too much salt in our diet. Hogwash and horse-spit. The problem is we're getting too much *artificial* salt in our systems. Sodium chloride is a manufacturing chemical. It is not natural salt. Got a container of Morton's? Chuck it. What you want comes in two types. There is real mineral salt mined from caves – it is pinkish and often clumps together. It is loaded with trace minerals and nutrients. The other type is ocean salt. These come white but also tend to clump up. Clumping salt? Just shake the container. Natural salt clumps. Shake it, break it up, sprinkle. Before I am deluged with "Salt is bad," let me say right here, "No, it is not."

Salt is required by the body for the function of your nervous system and the healthy functioning of your thyroid. Salt deficiency can lead to death. What you want to do is get off all *processed* salt and use the unfiltered, unbleached and untreated salt direct from mother nature and God Himself. The only time you should avoid even the natural salt is a pre-existing condition exacerbated by sodium (such as swelling). Once the condition goes away, introduce tiny bits of salt. When your body has had a chance to heal itself, such as with swelling, you will need salt. Not a lot. Don't get hyper with the salt-shaker.

Pepper. Black ground pepper. Many might shrug, but pepper can be a very good aid in shedding fat. Not only that, it is an anti-oxidant. The component in black pepper that is your best friend is piperine. Piperine blocks the formation of new fat cells, stimulates the metabolism to burn fat cells and sets off a whole chain reaction of fat-blocking and fat burning processes[61].

Piperine simulates the enzymes of the pancreas that breakdown proteins, speeding up the digestive process. Both West and East have used pepper to treat constipation, diarrhea, relieve gas and help improve digestion. It can also dramatically increase absorption of selenium, vitamin B and beta-carotene as well as other nutrients.

There's that Vitamin B again. Wink wink.

Piperine also helps to increase endorphins in the brain (which helps reduce pain and improve mood) thereby acting as a natural anti-depressant and increasing brain functions.

Wow, all from pepper.

I will say here that there is not a single spice that you shouldn't be eating. Oregano, parsley, basil, cinnamon, thyme, curry – you want it all. To end spices, I want to point out one in particular, **turmeric**.

You can get egregiously huge bags of turmeric from the wholesaler online. I think I have enough turmeric to feed several generations of descendants in my house. Don't buy the 25# bag. Trust me, the 5# bag is more than enough. Turmeric contains a wide range of antioxidant, antiviral, antibacterial, antifungal, anticarcinogenic, antimutagenic and anti-inflammatory properties. It is also loaded with many healthy nutrients such as protein, dietary fiber, niacin, Vitamin C, Vitamin E, Vitamin K, sodium, potassium, calcium, copper, iron, magnesium and zinc.

- Turmeric prevents cancer and destroys existing cancer cells.
- It relieves arthritis
- It reduces inflammation
- Controls diabetes and aids in reversing it
- Reduces your blood LDL cholesterol levels (it cleans your arteries!)
- It boosts the immune system
- Speeds healing
- Increases the bile flow in breaking down dietary fat
- Prevents Alzheimer's and breaks down the amyloid plaques – possibly starting a reversal of Alheimer's (more study needs to be done on that)

63

- Turmeric improves digestion and helps relieve Irritable Bowel Syndrome.
- It reduces bloating and gas.
- It detoxifies the liver and prevents liver disease.

Wow, all from turmeric[62]. Buy it, eat it, get well. **However, there is a danger to turmeric!** Yes, there is. If you are on medication for diabetes (blood sugar levels) you absolutely must ask your doctor if the particular medications he has prescribed work well with turmeric. Most medications are helped by turmeric, but there is one that can prove deadly. Ask, ask, ask.

One very big cautionary note on spices. Don't go out and buy a pre-mix "flavoring" like Lowry's. If it's in your cupboard, dump it. Throw it away. Don't even sniff it or wave goodbye. Pre-mixed shakes like that contain MSG – which will make you fat.

Here's a little bit about **hot sauces**. I have been on a hunt and found only one single sauce that does not contain **sodium benzoate**. It is a preservative that is toxic, causes damage to your DNA, and causes cancer. It can lead to ADHD in children, asthma, hypertension... well, let's just say you don't want it. Sodium benzoate turns into benzene in the presence of Vitamin C in the body[63]. Read your labels and avoid anything with sodium benzoate – and not just hot sauces, but all foods. By the way, that one single hot sauce I found without sodium benzoate? Good old Tabasco sauce. The original recipe and the Buffalo flavor both do not contain sodium benzoate.

However, their Jalapeno flavor does. Again, read your labels.

Also in many hot sauces and other foods is **guar gum** or **xanthum gum**. These are thickening agents. **In the body, they are a terror**. The gums can cause physical obstructions of your gastro-intestinal tract. They also block your body from absorbing critical nutrients and substances. The gums also cause colon cancer[64, 65].

Toss all your hot sauces. There's only one so far that appears good enough to keep: original red Tabasco Sauce. There are only three ingredients: aged red peppers, salt and vinegar. Red Tabasco is safe. Read the labels on the other Tabascos – they may contain other ingredients.

Next chapter will be about **Acid Reflux** and **Garlic**.

CHAPTER 10

A short recap:

- Wheat – very bad. Don't eat, don't touch, don't even have memories of it
- Eggs – very good for you
- Grass-fed organic beef is great! Regular beef is very bad
- Coconut, avocado, and olive oils are the only oils you should use for cooking
- Don't char your meat
- Coffee is good for you, sparingly
- Avoid all ocean seafood.
- Eliminate as many estrogens from your food as possible
- Eat lots of broccoli - not done talking about broccoli, either
- Eliminate as much plastic as possible – plastic is estrogenic
- Never use a microwave
- Buy organic, but not from china

However, their Jalapeno flavor does. Again, read your labels.

Also in many hot sauces and other foods is **guar gum** or **xanthum gum**. These are thickening agents. **In the body, they are a terror**. The gums can cause physical obstructions of your gastro-intestinal tract. They also block your body from absorbing critical nutrients and substances. The gums also cause colon cancer[64, 65].

Toss all your hot sauces. There's only one so far that appears good enough to keep: original red Tabasco Sauce. There are only three ingredients: aged red peppers, salt and vinegar. Red Tabasco is safe. Read the labels on the other Tabascos – they may contain other ingredients.

Next chapter will be about **Acid Reflux** and **Garlic**.

CHAPTER 10

A short recap:

- Wheat – very bad. Don't eat, don't touch, don't even have memories of it
- Eggs – very good for you
- Grass-fed organic beef is great! Regular beef is very bad
- Coconut, avocado, and olive oils are the only oils you should use for cooking
- Don't char your meat
- Coffee is good for you, sparingly
- Avoid all ocean seafood.
- Eliminate as many estrogens from your food as possible
- Eat lots of broccoli - not done talking about broccoli, either
- Eliminate as much plastic as possible – plastic is estrogenic
- Never use a microwave
- Buy organic, but not from china

- Eat spinach both raw and lightly fried in a fatty oil (bacon grease, olive, coconut oils)
- Eat red potatoes and red onions for the most nutrient value
- Turmeric and pepper block the formation of fat and burn it away
- Newt Gingrich: "The future of money is health care."

Going to talk about **garlic** and **acid reflux**. I'm going to skim through garlic because most of you have probably already heard it all.

Garlic. If you aren't eating it because you can't stand the flavor, then I understand. However, there are some tricks to garlic that can reduce the bite and smell. Reduce, not eliminate. Garlic has the following benefits:

- contains an antioxidant compound that prevents clotting, preventing heart attacks and strokes
- stops the spread of skin cancer when applied topically
- a good source of selenium and Vitamin C – protecting against colon cancer and even stopping it
- protects against ulcers and stomach cancer
- cooking it with your meat reduces the carcinogens if you do happen to char your meat

- the allicin from eating garlic promotes weight loss (more on that in a minute)
- lowers blood pressure
- lowers LDL (bad) cholesterol while raising HDL (good) cholesterol
- reduces the carcinogenic effects of asbestos exposure
- relieves arthritis
- reduces inflammation
- due to its antibacterial and antiviral properties, it wards against the flu and the cold
- prevents tuberculosis
- kills leukemia
- is a good source of Vitamin... yep, you guessed it, B6
- it is an effective anti-fungal agent for treating yeast infections, vaginitis, and athlete's foot
- protects the body from the ravages of diabetes

Here's something to consider about allicin and taking garlic supplements and preparing garlic. Garlic does not contain allicin, but rather allinin. Cutting the garlic and letting it sit for ten minutes or so activates the enzymes and converts allinin to allicin. Supplements are almost worthless for allicin because the process has fairly much destroyed the garlic.

So you want to eat your garlic raw, if you can – mix it into anything crushed, sliced, whatever. If you cook it, try not to cook it too long as cooking generally destroys Vitamin content. However you eat it, raw or cooked, remember to slice it and let it sit in the open air for a good ten minutes to activate the allicin.

Acid reflux. Or heartburn. Indigestion. Let's lump all that together because they're all interrelated. The garbage we have been eating, the gums, the glutens, the microwaved food have all caused damage to our digestive system. This becomes more serious over time as parts of our system just give up. This leads to acid reflux and an ever-worsening condition that can lead to burned and even collapsed esophagus.

Let me insert the fact that your dear author suffered from nightly heartburn. I woke up gagging every single night, that acid burn choking me and causing around two hours of sleepless throat clearing before I could finally go back to sleep. The most common advice I heard? Pop some antacid for immediate relief and prop up your pillow so you're in a sitting position. Great – nothing like advice that does nothing to cure it.

Cure? Yep. Cure. No pills, but your doctor won't want to tell you how to cure it – there's no money in a cure. Instead, your doctor will tell you how to treat it.

Do you want a cure? Or a lifelong treatment plan?

And guess what? Your dear author found the cure. 100% cure. No gimmicks, no bullshit. No weird tricks.

Acid reflux is serious. However, **it is not a disease**. It is a condition and so easily reversible, no matter what stage of this condition you are at. A disease? Please. The medical and pharmaceutical establishments want you to believe that because there is huge money in treating it. What they don't want you to know is the real cause behind acid reflux and how simple and easy it is to cure it. Disease? I can't scoff enough at the misnomer. It is not communicable, nor a virus that preys upon a weakened immune system. It is not a disease. Acid reflux is a *condition* brought on by diet. But let me tell you how this just gets worse and worse no matter what you try. Most of us remember "plop plop fizz fizz, oh what a relief it is." What a stupid little song that has done nothing but helped perpetuate total misery. We think," too much stomach acid, it's coming up – take an antacid." Some people pop Tums every night and the company even brags that it is fortified with nutrients.

What a load of crap.

Here's the skinny on Acid Reflux. That heartburn you feel? It's not too much acid, **it is too little**[66]. Don't stop reading. You will not hear that from your doctor. Antacids make the problem worse the next day, even with temporary relief the night before. Prescription pills to reduce acid guarantees to completely destroy your digestive system as your body makes less and less digestive acid and eventually fails completely. Here's the why and how: when your stomach does not have enough acid (because of the garbage with which you've been destroying your system), the food sits in the stomach. What happens is that lump of undigested food pushes the acid up the open esophagus. In a healthy system, your stomach registers the adequate level of acid and there is a sphincter at the opening of your stomach that clamps shut. You can stand on your head and nothing comes up.

So when your stomach does not have enough acid to digest what you gagged down, that sphincter remains open and you have another night of pain. It's as simple as that. It really is. No disease.

There is a simple, easy, totally ridiculously stupidly easy remedy (did I say stupid enough?): increase your stomach acid and feel that sphincter snap shut – it will, believe me. Take two tablespoons of extra virgin olive oil[67] every single night about two hours before going to bed, or sometime after your last meal of the day. The olive oil soothes your throat, causes instant acid creation in your stomach and you will feel slightly uncomfortable for about 15 minutes, maybe – while the oil is making acid. Then suddenly all discomfort will vanish. *You will feel that sphincter clamp – hard - shut and stay shut.* You will be able to sleep without taking antacids.

Takes time for your digestive system to heal itself.

Took about a month for me before I stopped the nightly olive oil. Some nights I had to take a second dosage. I have not had acid reflux except about once a year the first two years. I had this weird cold once each year and a bit of acid reflux, though nowhere near as bad as before. Even olive oil didn't stop it. The last once-a-year odd reflux I had was three years ago. Now? I sleep all night with not a hint of indigestion. From every night, painfully, never again. Would you like to sleep peacefully at night without gagging up acid? Without having to Tums it up every single night? Cure it completely? Olive oil.

Here's a story typical of people not wanting to learn anything – such as an acid reflux cure. I met a butcher at Safeway. He had acid reflux – really bad. I had just solved my condition several months before. I figured he wouldn't want to hear why olive oil worked, so I just told him the remedy. His condition had been worsening and worsening. He went through bottles and bottles of Tums. Finally he was on prescriptions **and** having to take more Tums on top of the prescriptions. I told him the remedy. Pestered him every week for two months: "Did you try it?"

Finally I told him why it worked. He was horrified. "More acid? No way." He went home, told his wife who was a nurse. The next week he said, "I told my wife about it and she said she had never heard of such nonsense and to not listen to anything you have to say." I tried to tell him to have his wife ask the doctor but he turned his back on me. I haven't spoken to him since.

Some people don't want to be helped and they don't want to help themselves. They just want a pill – even if it makes it worse.

I don't mean to end the chapter on something sounding so depressing, but we can be sure that one man, indicative of so many others, is keeping the antacid and pharmaceutical industries fat, wealthy, and so very happy.

Next chapter, **MSGs** and **High Fructose Corn Syrup**.

CHAPTER 11

A short recap:

- Wheat – very bad. Don't eat, don't touch, don't even have memories of it
- Eggs – very good for you
- Grass-fed organic beef is great! Regular beef is very bad
- Coconut, avocado, and olive oils are the only oils you should use for cooking
- Don't char your meat
- Coffee is good for you, sparingly
- Avoid all ocean seafood
- Eliminate as many estrogens from your food as possible
- Eat lots of broccoli - not done talking about broccoli, either
- Eliminate as much plastic as possible – plastic is estrogenic
- Never use a microwave
- Buy organic, but not from china

- Eat spinach both raw and lightly fried in a fatty oil (bacon grease, olive, coconut oils)
- Eat red potatoes and red onions for the most nutrient value
- Turmeric and pepper block the formation of fat and burn it away
- Garlic is a health wonder. Slice it 10 minutes before eating
- Acid Reflux is not a disease and easily curable with olive oil
- Newt Gingrich: "The future of money is health care."

This chapter is about **MSG** and **High Fructose Corn Syrup**. I know, I know, you all already know they're bad. But there are some very disturbing things about them that FOX or CNN won't tell you and the FDA continues to wink and look the other way while these toxins are put in your food.

MSG – Monosodium Glutamate is passed off as safe because glutamates naturally occur in foods and our bodies, but the MSG we eat today is an industrial fermentation of chemicals and no longer derived from plant sources (seaweed). MSG in our food is nothing close to "natural."

But many respected doctors, a prominent neurosurgeon[68] and several double-blind studies and one direct experiment have shown MSG can cause the following[69]:

- headaches
- chest pain

- heart palpitations
- nausea/vomiting
- difficulty breathing
- nervous system damage
- sleep disorders
- bipolar – mood swings
- chronic fatigue
- ADD, ADHD, Rage
- brain damage
- radical hormonal fluctuations
- kills your retinas
- causes obesity even in small amounts – specifically used to make labrats fat – **really fat**

A bit about that last point. MSG is an excitotoxin[70]. You cannot avoid its effects. In addition to all these wonderful profit incentives for your doctor, MSG is particularly addicting. Yes, food with MSG in it will make you fat, period, and no amount of "moderation" will stop it.

Don't ever eat it. Period.

Here's what you probably don't know.

MSG is allowed to be labeled by those crooks in Washington under the following disguised names:

- **monopotassium glutamate**
- **glutamate**
- **glutamic acid**
- **gelatin**
- **calcium caseinate**
- **hydrolyzed vegetable protein**

- **textured protein**
- **autolyzed plant protein**
- **hydrolyzed plant protein**
- **yeast extract glutamate**
- **yeast food or yeast nutrient**
- **sodium caseinate**
- **autolyzed yeast**

The following ingredients are made with MSG and the government does not require food manufacturers to label MSG as an ingredient when used with the following:

- **malted barley (flavor)**
- **barley malt**
- **malt extract of flavoring**
- **maltodextrin**
- **caramel flavoring (coloring)**
- **stock**
- **broth**
- **bouillon**
- **carrageenan**
- **whey protein or whey**
- **whey protein isolate or concentrate**
- **pectin**
- **protease**
- **protease enzymes**
- **flavors**   << Look, notice, understand
- **flavoring** << Look, notice, understand
- **natural chicken, beef or pork flavoring**

- **seasonings (if it is salt or pepper, or similar, they have to list it by law.)**
- **soy sauces or extract**
- **soy protein**
- **soy protein isolate or concentrate**
- **cornstarch**
- **flowing agents**
- **white rice or oat protein**
- **protein fortified anything**
- **enzyme modified anything**
- **ultra-pasteurized anything**
- **fermented anything**
- **annatto** - in almost all cheeses
- **spices** << Look, notice, understand
- **gums**
- **lipolyzed, modified, or conditioners**

Now, go down any aisle of the grocery store and pick up a box of "Heart Healthy" "All Natural" crap and see it for what it is. It will be full of fat-making MSGs.

High Fructose Corn Syrup. Deadly stuff. More deadly than you think. Basically, it is concentrated genetically modified corn sugar. There is a big push to bribe congress into letting the food companies hide the HFCS labeling under just "sweetener" or "corn sugar."

Here's what it does[71]:

- **causes obesity, fast, super-fast**
- **causes cancer**

- **causes heart disease**
- **causes kidney disease**
- **causes liver disease**
- **promotes kidney stones**
- **promotes gout**
- **magnifies the glycation end products in your body (you age faster)**

Sound fun? Your doctor loves it. The food and medical industries are making a killing off of killing you. But you would think we should get a hearty thanks from the food and medical industries – owned by certain globalists – but we don't. Nope. They think we're stupid. They think we are pathetically, retardedly stupid. Their goal is to kill as many people as possible while stealing their wealth through long deaths. Bill Gates and his "we'll reduce the population through vaccines[72]" and America signing Codex Alimentarius[73], which calls for a world population of 500 million[74]. Tinfoil? Then why did America sign it?

Know what's worse? Russian scientists found that HFCS destroyed the fertility in mice so that by the third generation the offspring were completely, irreversibly sterile[75]. We're shoveling this stuff down our kids' throats. I'm sure they'll thank us.

"But wait," you say. "We're stronger than mice." That's a popular myth. We are actually more susceptible to food effects than rodents[76] and far more susceptible than monkeys.

Hey, I'll make you a bet right here. Go pick up that colorful frozen food box that claims to be diet, claims to be "all natural," and claims to be "heart healthy." If you don't find at least three obesity-causing, health-destroying ingredients, I'll slink off quietly and not write about food again.

Next chapter will be about **soy** and **grocery shopping** in general.

CHAPTER 12

A short recap:

- Wheat – very bad. Don't eat, don't touch, don't even have memories of it
- Eggs – very good for you
- Grass-fed organic beef is great! Regular beef is very bad
- Coconut, avocado, and olive oils are the only oils you should use for cooking
- Don't char your meat
- Coffee is good for you, sparingly
- Avoid all ocean seafood
- Eliminate as many estrogens from your food as possible
- Eat lots of broccoli - not done talking about broccoli, either
- Eliminate as much plastic as possible – plastic is estrogenic
- Never use a microwave
- Buy organic, but not from china

- Eat spinach both raw and lightly fried in a fatty oil (bacon grease, olive, coconut oils)
- Eat red potatoes and red onions for the most nutrient value
- Turmeric and pepper block the formation of fat and burn it away
- Garlic is a health wonder. Slice it 10 minutes before eating
- Acid Reflux is not a disease and easily curable with olive oil
- Avoid all High Fructose Corn Syrup, all the time
- Avoid all MSGs ("flavorings," "spices," annatto, others)
- Newt Gingrich: "The future of money is health care."

Going to cover **Soy** and **Grocery Shopping** in this one. I touched on soy earlier but there is a huge misinformation campaign being run by the Big Food Monies of which we need to be aware. I'm going to touch on **Lotions**, too, but I will have to cover that more fully in the following chapter.

Soy. Up until about twenty years ago, soy was considered a weed. Yes, that's correct. The Big Monies want you to believe it has been eaten for thousands of years. That's the partial truth. It has not been eaten for thousands of years in the genetically modified form it is now. It has also never been eaten in history before it was genetically modified unless it first went through a detoxification process we know as fermenting. Fermenting is basically controlled rot. The toxins, through rotting, are turned into beneficial enzymes and nutrients. Only the Japanese did it.

That's right, Farmer Billy-Joe and his wife Ethel and their family of thirty-two kids in the 1700s in America did not eat soy. They *eradicated* it. Why? Because a soybean is toxic[77]. Today? Big Monies want you to believe it's healthy[78] – paid for by the mega-soybean growers. Sure, about as healthy as rat poison. You only unlock the nutrients in soy through fermentation and guess what? Our lovely kill-us-all politicians have decreed that such fermentation of soy is unavailable in the United States. In other words, move to Japan if you want to eat healthy, fermented soy.

Here's what soy does:

- **THE** most estrogenic food you can eat
- causes obesity
- **THE** largest contributor to inflammation that stores deadly toxins in your tissues
- causes allergies
- causes breast cancer
- causes uterine cancer
- causes infertility
- low or no libido
- shrinking male... parts
- **destroys** your thyroid
- blocks the digestion of protein, leading to thinning hair, weak bones

- promotes pancreatic cancer

Think a minute. There has been a stupidly enormous explosion in these maladies and deaths due to them since Big Monies pushed soy into our diet twenty years ago.

Want to know how deadly soy is? One bottle of infant soy formula has the estrogenic equivalent of giving your baby **four birth control pills**[78]. Do not ever feed soy to a child! Would any of you really give a baby four birth control pills for every meal? They throw you in prison for that kind of stuff, but the Big Monies get away with it pushing soy milk for babies.

Soy = NO. Ever. Do not touch it. *Do not even put it on your skin in **lotion** form.* Your skin absorbs anything you put on it and whatever you put on your skin eventually gets into your bloodstream – see the footnotes[79]. No soy is good. Not raw, not organic, not diet, not "healthy," not "in moderation," *not any kind.*

Don't believe Big Monies – their only interest is in you buying for their profits.

Grocery Shopping. There was a term I heard one day and it made just a ton of sense. If you go to the grocery store and "**shop the perimeter**" you will be far healthier as time goes by. Then I understood: the edges of the store contain your milks, cheeses, butters, eggs, meats, hams, fruits and vegetables. The center of the store contains all the pre-made packaged crap that is basically just a quick way to get you to eat five or six (at least) different forms of MSG or High Fructose Corn Syrup. The frozen aisle is the worst.

Why buy frozen? Buy fresh and freeze it yourself. We can't really be that lazy, can we? Frozen foods all contain MSG and/or soy. I spent time standing with my lovely wife (also my editor) going over many frozen foods about a year and a half ago. Yes, I grocery shop and no grocery shopping is done without me – of course, I also do all the cooking. Cheryl cleans, I cook: it works out. So anyway, we're standing there looking at deep fried fish (GM soy, GM wheat, MSG all over the place), the frozen waffles (ugh soy soy soy and some MSG to make it addictive), the Hot Pockets (not a single healthy ingredient), the frozen pizzas (soy, wheat, glutens, sugars, HFCS, maltodextrin), and then we looked at the frozen meats (glazes all contained MSG and many contained maltodextrin). What a total waste of time - except as an educational tool.

We spent extra time reading the labels of "Healthy This" and "Smart Choice That." We even picked up some "diet" foods and read those labels. All packed and crammed full of soy, maltodextrin, HFCS, flavorings, spices (MSG), and other crap you just cannot eat without causing cancer and obesity and a whole host of really bad stuff that makes Big Monies giggle with glee. The so-called "diet" foods were the worst.

The cereal aisle and chips and crackers are even worse. "Organic" does not mean "soy-free" or "canola-free." Often, the box brags about having a wonderful organic toxin that will have you suffering at the end of your life, whimpering in bed as someone else has to wipe your butt. Not for me, thanks.

Look, everyone has to die. Eating organic won't make you immortal, but it comes down to how you want to die. People used to keel over or die in their sleep. Pretty fast, pretty sudden. Long drawn out illnesses and diseases were not the norm. But now? Death is primarily a long drawn out hospital stay, in pain, suffering endlessly while they bilk your family of all their money. And that's the whole point behind all of these food toxins they are shoving down your throats. It's the whole Codex Alimentarius with America leading the way trying to reduce the global population down to 500 million and making huge profits while doing it!

"Quick" and "easy" food prepared for you is not food. Don't touch it. Quick and easy is organic celery with some 100% peanut butter on it (no sugars). Quick and easy is some raw mushrooms or an organic apple or organic orange. Quick and easy is a few slices of uncured ham (yum!) with some pure cheese. Quick and easy is grabbing a handful of raw, organic spinach and munching away. Quick and easy is a handful of walnuts.

Here's a grocery-trick about walnuts. The grocery store will have two places for walnuts and guess what? They charge more for the same weight depending on where you pick up that package! The baking aisle usually has your more expensive walnuts. Your perimeter will have walnuts that are cheaper by the pound. When they're $7 per pound and they charge another dollar an aisle over, you're smart to avoid the baking aisle for walnuts.

Microwaved popcorn or pizza is just pure stupidity, period, no excuse.

Most canned foods contain a BPA liner – remember my chapter on BPA? Most of the Big Monies companies use it and gladly. They want to kill us off, remember? Avoid the big-name canned foods. Even if not for the BPA liners, the food inside is packed with sugars, MSGs, gums, glutens, maltodextrins, high fructose corn syrup and other garbage. Soups are the worst – *even organic soups*. I have yet to find a real organic soup that does not contain at least one MSG ("natural flavorings" or "natural spices"). Sauces are as bad as soups and maybe worse. Those packages all ready to add milk or water? Pure poison.

It doesn't really take all that much time to put a pan on the stove and go do something while your food cooks.

I will be presenting a typical range of menu items I have found safe and healthy to eat later. There isn't much and it's not like going to a restaurant and being able to choose from forty-nine pages of menu. In fact, at first, it is depressing how small our healthy choices are. But the alternative is that long, suffering death...

Next chapter I will talk about **lotions** and **Diet Sodas**.

CHAPTER 13

A short recap:

- Wheat – very bad. Don't eat, don't touch, don't even have memories of it
- Eggs – very good for you
- Grass-fed organic beef is great! Regular beef is very bad
- Coconut, avocado, and olive oils are the only oils you should use for cooking.
- Don't char your meat
- Coffee is good for you, sparingly
- Avoid all ocean seafood
- Eliminate as many estrogens from your food as possible
- Eat lots of broccoli - not done talking about broccoli, either
- Eliminate as much plastic as possible – plastic is estrogenic
- Never use a microwave
- Buy organic, but not from china

- Eat spinach both raw and lightly fried in a fatty oil (bacon grease, olive, coconut oils)
- Eat red potatoes and red onions for the most nutrient value
- Turmeric and pepper block the formation of fat and burn it away
- Garlic is a health wonder. Slice it 10 minutes before eating
- Acid Reflux is not a disease and easily curable with olive oil
- Avoid all High Fructose Corn Syrup, all the time
- Avoid all MSGs ("flavorings," "spices," annatto, others)
- Avoid all soy, avoid all soy, and avoid all soy
- Shop the perimeter of your grocery store and read the labels!
- Newt Gingrich: "The future of money is health care."

This chapter will be **lotions** and **diet sodas**. This will also touch back on **olive oil** and **frying pans**. You'll see how the thread weaves. Imagine it also leading to make-up and even sexual lubricants (gasp!).
Oh brother.

Lotions. There are so few lotions worth buying that it is easier to avoid them entirely. Here's why: most contain agents that cause a silky smooth feeling. Those are parabens. There's a whole family of parabens. Methyl Paraben, Ethyl Paraben, Fred Paraben and Ricky and Lucy Paraben. Sure, that's a bit of a joke, but any kind of paraben is extremely bad to be putting on your skin[80]. Parabens soak into your pores and eventually enter your bloodstream. Guess what? Parabens are highly estrogenic, and these are chemical parabens, not naturally occurring parabens in certain foods. They:

- DESTROY your thyroid
- cause ovarian cancer
- cause breast cancer
- cause skin cancer
- damage your hypothalmus
- cause damage and shrinkage in male... parts
- promotes the formation of cancer cells everywhere in the body

Before you swish this information away with your hand, consider that drinking the stuff is considered toxic, call your doctor, warning label hysteria and paramedics and all that. Guess what? You absorb many times more into your bloodstream rubbing it on your skin *than drinking it*. Parabens are found in **lotions, shampoos, sexual lubricants,** and **make-up**. Read your labels, it is possible to find replacements for all of those.

Basically it boils down to this for lotions. **Never** put anything onto your body you cannot drink or eat. Need moisturizer? There is no better moisturizer than wetting your skin with filtered water and applying a rub of **olive oil** – or something odorless like avocado oil. You can buy and use the "light" olive oils for those – they don't have the smell of extra-virgin olive oil. Being that the olive oil will soak into the skin, you might even be helping your body reduce bad cholesterol, lower your blood pressure, and improve overall cardiovascular health in a minute way.

"Minute way" brings up another point. Many of the doctors[81] I read all agreed that these toxic substances even in the most minute amounts had a negative effect on the body. One might argue, "Oh, a little bit of this won't hurt." Yes it will! "Well, I can't go without my favorite lotion with its lavender fragrance." You mean you can't go without your breast cancer? Fragrance is a whole other topic. I will need to cover that next email. But even the most minute amount of these toxins accumulates in the body, working with all the other toxins from other substances, foods, fragrances, soaps, emissions and whew – just everything – to produce a never-ending supply of cancer direct to you. Free shipping!

Diet Sodas. I used to drink 12+ cans of it a day. Glad I quit. But let me briefly mention regular soda. Regular soda is in no way good for you or better than diet sodas – don't believe the Big Monies that regular soda sweetened with "fruit sugar" is better for you. That's a derivative, genetically modified and often mixed with HFCS. Don't fall for the lie! Diet soda, on the other hand, is even worse than regular soda. Go figure. The aspartame was originally developed by the military as a chemical weapon[82]. That's right, a Weapon of Mass Destruction. I know it sounds stupid, but it's true. The military dropped it because it killed too slowly. Remember Donald Rumsfeld, the Military Chief of Staff? Some time ago, he pushed the FDA to get it passed as safe. He was, at that particular time, also the CEO of the pharmacidal company that produced it. Aspartame is in **Nutrasweet**, **Equal**, and others. Check your labels. But what aspartame does is sick enough as it is[83]:

- Causes headaches
- Causes brain tumors
- Causes brain lesions
- Causes lymphoma
- Memory loss
- Causes leukemia
- DESTROYS your nervous system

Also in most sodas is phenylalinine. It is a neurotoxin. It will work with aspartame to enhance the destruction of your nervous system[84]. It will also bring a huge smile to Donald Rumsfeld's face and the obesity of his wallet.

Stevia is a safe sweetener alternative, and natural. Xylitol is safe but only if it comes from Finland! Non-Finnish sources are a chemical recreation and not very well-received by the digestive tract. Xylitol comes originally from the Finnish Birch tree. Since its discovery, Xylitol can now be made chemically from just about anything. American Xylitol is made from corn. That's right, good old GM corn. Read your labels and avoid Xylitol unless you are sure it comes from Finland. In fact, other than Stevia and Finnish Xylitol, avoid all "sugar alcohols" such as maltitol, sorbitol, (anything ending with "itol"). All of those sugar alcohols are chemically produced and not digestible by the body – causing cramps, bloating, and possible digestive tract maladies such as IBS and others.

There is one more factor to consider about soda consumption and this is going to throw me back to frying pans. I know, I know, but be patient. Sodas and many drinks are "bottled" in **aluminum** cans. Should we really be drinking liquids from aluminum cans? Aluminum is present in many maladies, though there has not yet been a firm connection between it and cancer. There is strong evidence, but nothing yet proven. Aluminum accumulates in the kidneys, brain, lungs, liver, bladder, and thyroid where it competes with calcium for absorption and can affect skeletal mineralization. In infants, this can slow growth. Animal models have linked aluminum exposure to mental impairments[85]. Aluminum shows up in Alzheimers, Parkinsons, many cancers (brain, breast, kidney, bone, the list goes on), brain disorders, and neurological disorders.

You think, wait a minute, I'm not eating it. Oh yes, you are. The metal leeches into everything it contains. Aluminum is thus consumed with your sodas or other drinks from aluminum cans. Don't shake your head. Back in history, tomatoes used to be considered poisonous. Why? Because they would be served with all the other food on lead plates[86]. But the acids from a tomato worked with the lead and gave an instant dose of lead-poisoning to the eater. They ate the tomato, not the plate. That now brings up cooking pans again. Many people use aluminum cookware.

Heating anything allows the more rapid dispersal of whatever it is. Iron cookware releases more iron into the food (good for women, bad for men) when it is heated. Likewise aluminum. Heat aluminum and you're getting some extra-heavy and constant doses of a metal your body does not need and is quite unhealthy. Replace it all with stainless steel and don't look back. Stainless steel works just fine. Aluminum foil? No-no. I don't think they even make tin foil anymore.

Next chapter: **Fragrances** and **Soaps**. I still intend to get back to broccoli... but I will do it when I talk about apples.

CHAPTER 14

A short recap:

- Wheat – very bad. Don't eat, don't touch, don't even have memories of it.
- Eggs – very good for you.
- Grass-fed organic beef is great! Regular beef is very bad.
- Coconut, avocado, and olive oils are the only oils you should use for cooking.
- Don't char your meat.
- Coffee is good for you, sparingly.
- Avoid all ocean seafood.
- Eliminate as many estrogens from your food as possible
- Eat lots of broccoli - not done talking about broccoli, either
- Eliminate as much plastic as possible – plastic is estrogenic
- Never use a microwave

- Buy organic, but not from china
- Eat spinach both raw and lightly fried in a fatty oil (bacon grease, olive, coconut oils)
- Eat red potatoes and red onions for the most nutrient value
- Turmeric and pepper block the formation of fat and burn it away
- Garlic is a health wonder. Slice it 10 minutes before eating
- Acid Reflux is not a disease and easily curable with olive oil
- Avoid all High Fructose Corn Syrup, all the time
- Avoid all MSGs ("flavorings," "spices," annatto, others)
- Avoid all soy, avoid all soy, and avoid all soy
- Shop the perimeter of your grocery store and read the labels!
- Lotions – if you can't eat it, don't use it
- Avoid all sodas both regular and diet
- Ditch all your aluminum in the trash
- Newt Gingrich: "The future of money is health care."

Going to talk about **fragrances** and **soaps** and touch on **shampoos**. I know this is off food, but it needs to be said because this is yet another piece in the multi-part puzzle of obesity and sickness.

Fragrances. They're in practically everything. We always like to have pleasant smells around, without a doubt. From laundry detergent to air fresheners to perfumes. The problem is, the vast majority of fragrances aren't something natural like lavender oil or petunia oil. Nearly all fragrances are chemically constructed in a lab and the chemicals are toxic to the body[87].

These chemicals are found in artificially scented air fresheners, soaps, detergents and cleaners, deodorants, lotions, perfumes and other common products.

Many of the chemicals used to formulate certain aromas are actually petrochemicals. Petrochemicals are derived from natural gas and petroleum. Benzene, toluene, xylenes, and methanol are some of the common petrochemicals used in these aromatic concoctions. About 95% of the "fragrances" are these deadly toxins. Just to take, for instance, benzene:

- causes cancer
- causes leukemia
- destroys your bone marrow
- causes anemia
- creates immune deficiencies
- the fumes damage your cornea
- putting it on your skin can result in dermatitis and blistering

That's just one part of the chemical toxin we call "fragrance." Fragrances are also high in

phthalates, remember them? Short reminder.
Phthaltes:

- are endocrine disruptors, destroying hormonal balance
- cause cancer
- cause infertility
- cause birth defects
- cause shrinkage of male... parts
- destroys testosterone
- causes ADHD

So here's the best advice on fragrances. Stop wearing perfumes, buy only unscented laundry detergent. Unscented fabric softener. Stop buying "air fresheners," especially those insidious little devices that plug into the wall and spit toxins into the air especially for your pleasure and later the doctor's pleasure. Don't buy incense unless it comes from India or Tibet or some place that still makes genuine sandalwood or the like. Don't use "scented" anything. If you really think you must wear perfume, at least spray the toxin on your clothes instead of on your skin. You'll still be a walking toxin-zombie to yourself and everyone around you but at least you limit direct skin exposure for yourself.

More advice: don't believe those ridiculous Television commercials where a woman picks up her clean laundry and inhales with an orgasmic look across her features. Forget the aroma of detergents; just make sure your clothes are clean.

Here's a story. I had this severe leg-itching problem around my ankles for several years. Even bought a vegetable brush and I would scratch endlessly. My ankles were a bloody mess every day. At night, I would use my toenails to dig in. Even bought a second hard-plastic tile scrub brush for nighttime itching relief. I gouged at my ankles and shin and often the brush came away bloody. Then I learned about fragrances. Switched to unscented detergent with no sodium lauryl sulfate and all the itching vanished. What a relief. I still have the brushes, but using them is a dim memory.

That brings up **shampoos**. Nearly all shampoos contain sodium lauryl sulfate among other toxic ingredients[88]. It is the cleaning agent that foams in your shampoos and soaps, in toothpastes and make-up. Problem is, the stuff soaks through your pores and here's a list of what that wonderful chemical does to you:

- possibly a carcinogen by itself
- reacts with other chemicals to form nitrosamines in your tissues (remember charred meat?) and that *does* cause cancer
- damages your liver and kidneys
- causes nervous system damage
- causes hair loss

Sodium lauryl sulfate might be made from coconuts, but the chemical process of refinement includes dioxane and ethylene oxide. Those do cause cancer. A better alternative, though still somewhat of an irritant, is sodium laureth sulfate. This version does not use cancer-causing chemicals in refinement and is too large to be absorbed by the skin. Also available is the large-molecule sodium lauryl sulfoacetate – too large to penetrate the skin. For shampoo, there are growing choices and some boast SLS-free labels. Here's a great one for a fantastic price: Kirkland's Professional Salon Formula Moisture Shampoo. Comes in a tall, purple, squarish bottle and runs around $12 and you get a lot of it. Lasts for months. Incidentally, produced and distributed to salons in smaller bottles going for outrageous prices. You can find the Kirkland brand at the club stores like Price, Costco, Three Bears in Montana... ha.

SLS is also in your **hand soaps**. If your hand soap comes in a pump bottle, just throw it away. Buy bars of Ivory or Kirk's Castile.

SLS is also in your **toothpaste**. If you're using Crest or Aim or some stupid big brand name like that still even after knowing fluoride is a neurotoxin[89], throw those away, too.

There is no better toothpaste than a swish of hydrogen peroxide followed by dipping a wet toothbrush in good old **Baking Soda**.

Pick up your deodorant and read the ingredients. You'll get sick. Breast cancer on the rise? But of course those cancerous tissues all contain large amounts of aluminum. Guess what the primary ingredient of deodorant is for blocking odor? Mmm hmm. Aluminum. And you're applying that right next to fatty tissues where it accumulates[90]. It's easy to find scoffers on the internet. They claim worries amount to nothing and to keep using and/or eating whatever it is causing concern. They claim "There are no studies confirming…" Do you want to risk your health on someone's opinion? I prefer hard science. Here's the ugly truth about deodorants. They aren't really deodorants. Odor is caused by bacteria. Odor does not come from your body. Moisture comes out of your body and reacts with bacteria in the air and on your clothing. A deodorant clogs your pores and masks the odor. It also permanently binds odor into your clothing. Clean? Put on a previously worn shirt when you used deodorant and even after laundering you will stink in minutes. Your shirt gave you the odor.

Here's the advice on deodorant. Throw it away! But, you will also have to replace your shirts, t-shirts, blouses, and probably even your bras. Wear a cotton t-shirt under everything. Cotton allows your body to perspire if it needs to but keeps you cool and mostly dry. Unless you're exercising or something. This is what to use for a real deodorant – since bacteria is the cause of your odor, you want to kill the bacteria. KILL IT, not mask it. Easiest way is Isopropyl Rubbing Alcohol. However, that product is made from petroleum and you certainly don't want to drink it. A better way is to simply go buy a big bottle of **Vodka**. Yes, vodka. It has no smell. Mix 1 part Vodka to 3 parts water. IF you can stand the initial smell of Apple Cider Vinegar, mix enough of that in to give a little color. The vinegar smell goes away in 2-3 minutes. I use a glass vinegar bottle with a sprayer top. I spray, apply, and I'm off for the day.

Vinegar aids in keeping the bacteria away. But, if you just can't stand the initial vinegar smell, straight vodka and water will do the trick. Might need to apply that twice a day, but the health benefits should be plain to see. I will talk more about vodka and drinking at the end of the book.

I brought these non-food topics up because of the hormonal disruptions they cause. They force your body to build estrogenic tissues which force more fat building and more and more. It is a never-ending fight when your body is geared to building fat – even if all you eat is a single Saltine per day.

Back to foods next chapter. **Broccoli**, finally, and I will begin talking about typical meals starting with **breakfast** and the dangers of **tomatoes**! Oh no!

CHAPTER 15

A short recap:

- Wheat – very bad. Don't eat, don't touch, don't even have memories of it
- Eggs – very good for you
- Grass-fed organic beef is great! Regular beef is very bad
- Coconut, avocado, and olive oils are the only oils you should use for cooking
- Don't char your meat
- Coffee is good for you, sparingly
- Avoid all ocean seafood.
- Eliminate as many estrogens from your food as possible
- Eat lots of broccoli - not done talking about broccoli, either
- Eliminate as much plastic as possible – plastic is estrogenic
- Never use a microwave
- Buy organic, but not from china

- Eat spinach both raw and lightly fried in a fatty oil (bacon grease, olive, coconut oils)
- Eat red potatoes and red onions for the most nutrient value
- Turmeric and pepper block the formation of fat and burn it away
- Garlic is a health wonder. Slice it 10 minutes before eating
- Acid Reflux is not a disease and easily curable with olive oil
- Avoid all High Fructose Corn Syrup, all the time
- Avoid all MSGs ("flavorings," "spices," annatto, others)
- Avoid all soy, avoid all soy, and avoid all soy
- Shop the perimeter of your grocery store and read the labels!
- Lotions – if you can't eat it, don't use it
- Avoid all sodas both regular and diet
- Ditch all your aluminum in the trash
- Newt Gingrich: "The future of money is health care."

Back to **broccoli** today, a breakfast **menu** and the danger of **tomatoes!**

First I want to say that although I have mentioned Gingrich and Rumsfeld, I am not a democrat. Neither am I a republican. Neither am I independent. In fact, I am apolitical. I think the whole

structure is rigged, phony, corrupt and designed to
entertain us. According to the constitution, we do not
elect the president and the electoral college does not
have to consider the public vote. Law. The last real
president we had was probably JFK. Look at his
policies and the hysterical types would be screaming
that JFK was an extreme right-wing radical Tea
Partier and dangerous for the country.

Enough of politics lest I feel the need to go
take another shower. Pure filth and scumbaggery.

Broccoli first. Buy organic if you can find it.
Wash it thoroughly in reverse osmosis filtered water.
Make sure any dust is removed (radioactive
Fukushima stuff). Here's what I left out before. You
buy this broccoli and most people cut the florets loose
and cook/eat those. Florets are the flowery head of
broccoli. The thing is, that's the most bitter part of the
vegetable. The stalks are the most flavorful and
usually the part people throw away. Don't throw away
the thick stalk you paid money for!

You might as well eat it and here's why: the
stalk is just as nutritious as the florets, if not more!
And tastier. The stalk as it thickens towards the base
becomes tougher. Some people skin them like
potatoes to remove the chewy skin. Leave the skin on.
In most fruits and veggies you're going to find most
of the nutrients in the skin or right underneath. Peel it
and you're going to remove the nutrients.

Instead, cut off about the bottom half inch of
the dried-out stalk and chuck it. Throw it at your cat.
Then slice what you want in thin slices off the stalk.
Fry that up lightly in coconut oil or olive oil (or both).

It makes a great topping for any omelet, scramble, or a side dish for breakfast lunch or dinner. It doesn't even need to be seasoned.

Potential breakfast items:

- Eggs, 2-3, any way you like them, but make sure the egg white is cooked through
- Bacon, don't char it
- Ham, if you cook it, don't char it Better to eat it uncooked.
- Oatmeal, unsweetened generally, or a touch of raw unfiltered honey
- Oatmeal O's cereal, unsweetened, or with a touch of honey or some fruit slices. Use only non-wheat O's
- Potatoes, lightly fried
- Fruit, fresh and organic

I like to pile my breakfast with protein and fat straight away. There is some scuttlebutt that what you eat as the first meal of the day conditions your body to metabolize that choice. So if you start the day with fruit, you're going to metabolize more sugar. If you eat fats, you metabolize more fats. I don't buy that and I think it's a crock of bull. So there. I rather just like feeling full and all the fats and fatty oils last me all the way to dinner with nothing more than an apple or some nuts or celery in between.

Egg breakfast scramble:

- ➢ Crack two eggs into a bowl and beat with fork
- ➢ Saute very lightly some white mushrooms and a good handful of organic spinach – the spinach shrinks considerably. Use extra virgin olive oil and a slice of butter
- ➢ Add eggs to the saute. Sprinkle turmeric into the cooking glob
- ➢ In your breakfast bowl, slice maybe ¼ cup of raw red onion. If you can stand it, ½ a cup
- ➢ Dump the cooked egg scramble on top of the onion.
- ➢ Douse as much black pepper onto the pile as you can stand. Pour it, don't sprinkle
- ➢ Grab a tissue because your nose will run.

While I am preparing all that, I sometimes have a sliced red potato frying in avocado and coconut oil. For a creamier texture, I add a slice of butter in with it to cook. If your fork melts into the potato, they're more than done. But you do want to cook them, never eat a potato raw. I put the slices on a plate when they are done cooking and sprinkle turmeric on each one. The turmeric will soak into the oil. Then I dose them with enough black pepper to choke two elephants. In other words, a lot of black pepper.

If you have followed my information in these chapters, you will note that I have just about filled my daily requirements for nutrients with that one simple meal. Not only that, with the addition of turmeric and black pepper, I am forcing my body to shed and eliminate estrogenic tissues and blocking any others from forming.

The danger of tomatoes! Oh noes! (screams)

Tomatoes are a fantastic fruit that should be eaten whenever you can. I love dumping a bunch of organic diced tomatoes on my beef or whatever I am having for dinner. Yum! But never, ever with eggs. Do not put tomatoes into your eggs. Might taste great but the tomatoes block your body from absorbing lutein and our primary source of lutein is going to be eggs.

Next chapter will be the depressingly small and shrinking **lunch** and **dinner** choices. And yes, it is very depressing.

CHAPTER 16

I'll dispense with the recap. I'll start with a short introduction to this chapter. There are so many factors that affect health – not just from what we eat, but the plastics and toxins in the fragrances and our environment.

If it seems as if every possible effort has been made to develop products and foods that increase estrogen and thus force us to be fat, then we are probably seeing the trees but just can't accept the forest. All the evidence is there from Bill Gates saying he wants to reduce the population using vaccines to the globalists bragging they want a population of 500 million worldwide[91]. Take a look online at "the Georgia Guidestones" - a monument erected by the globalists celebrating their goals of killing 95% of the world's population through whatever means necessary.

Lunch/Snacks

There are great choices here and all have some very positive benefits. If it comes in a box, it's not a snack, it's an attack on your system and all these little attacks add up.

Nuts: raw walnuts are awesome. Drop the bag of candied walnuts. Walnuts reduce plaque accumulation on your arteries, lower your bad cholesterol... in fact, I am going to go off on a small rant here.

Anyone who thinks you need overall low cholesterol either doesn't know what they are talking about or isn't telling you the whole truth. Cholesterol is required by the body for proper cell function, the processing of Vitamin D and hormonal balance. Is there a cholesterol level that is too high? Sure if you have a high level of LDL cholesterol. Cholesterol levels over 300? No problem – if your levels are predominantly HDL cholesterol. Reducing total cholesterol is as unhealthy as having high LDL cholesterol in the first place. If you are eating right, celebrate a high cholesterol level! High HDL cholesterol will not kill you.

Peanuts are great, too. Do not buy the toffee-covered nuts. You would totally destroy the health benefits with all the chemicals. Also, beware Planters Dry Roasted. Dry roasted nuts are fine but Planters comes chock full of colorings, flavorings, MSG, and cancer. Leave them alone. If you can get salted nuts with sea salt, those are fine. **Warning** about peanuts: they will make you very sleepy.

Cashews are wonderful and so are macadamias. Macadamias have a high fat content, but it is the kind of fat you want. No, macadamias will not make you fat – unless you buy the chocolate-coated ones.

Almonds are fantastic. Dry roasted with sea salt and nothing else, almonds make a great snack and are a rich source of vitamin E, calcium, phosphorous, iron and magnesium. They also contain zinc, selenium, copper and niacin. Compared to all other nuts, almonds are the most packed with nutrients and beneficial components. Hint: don't buy baking almonds. Not only are they incredibly hard on the teeth, but are more expensive in the baking aisle. Buy dry roasted from the nut aisle or perimeter of the store. Easier to chew and easier on the pocket book. **Warning** about almonds: they will make you sleepier than peanuts. But the sleepiness goes away after an hour. Perfect to grab a handful and then pass out for a nap. They are great before bed, too, as they will drop you into a nice deep sleep.

Sunflower seeds are really dicey. They are an excellent source of Vitamin E, Vitamin B1, Vitamin B6, manganese, copper, selenium, phosphorous, and folate. Also a fine source of antioxidants. But, pick up a typical package of shelled seeds and they're roasted in canola oil or corn oil or soy oil bad, bad bad. Very bad, drop the package. You have to buy your sunflower seeds still in the shell and pick the little things out the old fashioned way. Be careful of the ingredients. Some companies spray the outside of the shell with flavorings. **Warning**: eating a lot of them will give you gas. A lot of gas. You have been warned. Update: Safeway started carrying a sunflower seed without using soy or canola oil. Read your labels.

And really, any kind of raw or dry-roasted nut with sea salt is good.

Celery is also a great snack. Goes well with 100% peanut butter. Celery is an excellent source of vitamin C, fiber, folic acid, potassium, and vitamins B1 and B6. It is also a good source of vitamin B2 and calcium. **Warning**: celery will make you slightly sleepy.

White Mushrooms (or brown) are a fine snack eaten raw. Mushrooms provide health benefits that include relief from high cholesterol levels, breast cancer, prostate cancer, and diabetes. It also helps in weight loss, and increases the strength of your immune system.

Avocados are a super snack. Don't blink at the price. Avocados contain vitamins A, B, C, E, and K, iron, magnesium, folic acid, copper, fiber, protein, and potassium. Avocados also contain phytonutrients. Avocados contain 18 essential amino acids which can be used to form a complete protein. The health benefits are staggering. They promote cardiovascular health, boost your immune system, reduce inflammation, lowers LDL cholesterol while raising HDL cholesterol, regulates your blood pressure, lowers risk for all types of cancer, fights prostate cancer directly, increases your absorption of some nutrients by a factor of five, rich in antioxidants, prevents diabetes, regulates blood sugar, reverses insulin resistance, and is a good source of lutein that prevents cataracts and macular degeneration. Hint: remember tomatoes block your body's absorption of lutein. Try to eat the avocado separate from tomatoes. Remember to wash your avocados before you slice them open.

A good snack: **Guacamole!** But not made the normal way. Various recipes exist. Many use mayonnaise. Blech, soy, no, never. Here's mine: mash one avocado with 2 tablespoons of organic sour cream. Dump in a tablespoon of cayenne pepper and two or three teaspoons of black pepper. No salt. Grab a tissue, your nose will run. Eat by scooping with raw mushrooms or finding that ultra-rare product I am about to describe...

Corn Chips. If you must have a snack of the crunchy variety, it is possible to find corn chips that are Non-GMO, use sea salt and Non-GMO corn oil. But your search may take you to a couple different stores. They go good with beans or guacamole! However, remember that even Non-GMO corn is still high in Omega 6 fatty acids and you don't want to eat more than a few per day.

Pork Rinds! Yeah, that's right. Pork rinds are awesome. Pure fat of the good kind and you can scarf a whole bag and the fat will just melt off of you. Pork rinds are a source of several vitamins. Vitamin B12, riboflavin, niacin, thiamin are present and other vitamins occur in pork rinds in smaller quantities, including vitamin A, vitamin C, vitamin E, vitamin B6, and pantothenic acid. Pork rinds! Be careful of the super dark hard parts, I lost half a molar to one.

Bread. "But I thought you said bread was bad?" I did. Pay attention. Some bread can be found that contains only rice and simple ingredients. Be aware though, don't just grab the first rice bread you see. Most contain soy. Bad bad bad. If you can find a rice bread without soy or canola or other bad-dog chemicals, then these can make a great sandwich. First, rice bread is bland. Very bland. Throw your slices on the grill and fry them in butter and olive oil. Spread a thin layer of organic sour cream on them (or homemade mayonnaise), pile some fresh spinach, blob a bit of 100% mustard and put a slice of raw ham on it. Or you could go the hot route and fry that bread with slices of cheese on them and heat the ham next to them. Pile it up for a runny, gooey, delicious mess. Don't fall for the whole grain, multi-grain, 7-grain, 500-grain, "Bible" grain, or any of the other tricks they use to get you to buy GM wheat, soy and canola oils. Check your labels! One bad ingredient ruins it.

Avoid all packaged snacks otherwise. Beef jerky? Forget it. "Heart Healthy Diet Bars?" Don't make me giggle; it is unseemly that a man should giggle. Candies, cookies, pastries, ice cream, just forget it, okay? Pick one up and horrify yourself with the toxins and DNA-destroying crap in all of those.

Rice and **beans**, next chapter.

CHAPTER 17

This chapter adds another couple of foods to the acceptable list. **Rice** and **beans**.

Beans first. Don't buy canned beans. Only one brand that I know of (Safeway-brand cheapie refried) does not contain a list of MSGs, soy and canola oils. (Update: Safeway's brand now adds bad-dog ingredients but we have found some new organic canned providers. Check your labels.)

Remember, big name brands typically are poisoning you with addictive additives and because they get a wink and a nod from their former employees who now work at the FDA, they don't care if it destroys your health.

You would think that a food without all the additives would cost less, right? Rarely. Seems like they jack up the price faster the less ingredients.

Soak your own beans. Takes a day, minimum for beans like pintos and navy or white beans. Two days is better and three days is best. At three days, the bean water will smell like nine different flavors of toilet, so drain them off and pour fresh water for cooking. Why three days? Your beans will smell less as they cook and also produce less gas in your intestines. Supposedly. I won't stand by that claim although I would say there might be less gas at 3 days. It's not like it disappears and you can dance, frolicking in the flowers and all that.

Pinto beans are high in molydenum, folate, fiber, manganese and protein. They are a good source of Phosphorous, Vitamin B1, magnesium, potassium, and iron.

Black eyed peas are a good source of protein, fiber, folate, potassium, iron, manganese, and Vitamin A.

Boil on medium low for a few hours. Boiling retains almost all of the nutrients. Canned has almost no nutrients as they were depleted in the canning process. Pick a bean out every once in a while. When it looks as if it is beginning to shed skin, they're about done. They should be soft to the bite. Melt a cube of butter into it and mash for a runny bean soup. Or leave whole. The butter will help congeal everything together for leftover servings and gives a good flavor/texture.

Beans go good with beef as a mixture, with a decent amount of cayenne pepper to give it some kick. A tablespoon of onion powder or minced raw onion is good, too. Melt some cheese into the mixture and you have a very healthy way to get some vital nutrients into your body.

Rice: should only be bought as whole brown rice. Don't buy white rice, it is fairly devoid of nutrients. Except I understand Basmati White Rice is good and Basmati contains less arsenic than other forms of rice. Don't buy boxes of rice. No, no. Minute rice? Pointless. Take the time to get real rice, whole brown rice, and boil it up yourself. Takes about 45 minutes to boil up two handfuls of rice with 2 cups of water. The benefits to brown rice:

- reduces the risk of diabetes
- good source of natural fiber
- contains manganese
- contains selenium
- prevents weight gain
- lowers bad cholesterol
- raises good cholesterol
- protects against arterial plaque build-up
- helps prevent many types of cancer
- contains magnesium

Rice goes good with almost everything. Goes with beef, chicken, beans, beef hot dogs, and even alone with a good cut of broccoli mixed in for a veggie dinner. And also, soup!

I like to make my own **chicken soup**, which is so incredibly easy. Fry up a package of organic chicken in a half cup of extra-virgin olive oil. Add in a cube of butter. Cover and cook on medium low for about 10 minutes. When you uncover to check, your chicken should be white on the tops. Flip them over. Too much brown on the bottom means your temp was too high (so you know next time). As they are cooking on the flipside, take a couple of heavy steak knives and start slicing them up. I crosscut them with two knives and feel all manly doing it. Gives a good upper arm work-out. I suppose you could even dance while cutting, maybe to Barry Manilow. Just don't tell me about it. The chicken should be white on the inside. Don't mistake the pinkish juice for uncooked chicken. It's just juice. Reduce the heat to low. Slice up one to four cloves of garlic and let it sit for ten minutes. Sprinkle turmeric and curry on the chicken mess. Salt lightly. Dump in a couple tablespoons of cayenne pepper. Pour 2 cups of hot water into the pan. Crack two eggs into it and start beating them in the pan. This will make sort of like an egg-drop soup effect. Throw in the garlic and cover. Raise the heat slightly and wait five minutes. There's your chicken soup, and a very healthy one at that. Sometimes I add rice. There will be plenty of leftovers.

For more dinner suggestions:

- ➤ Fried chicken breasts or tenders heated with cheese so it melts, served over rice with or without spinach and/or sauted mushrooms.
- ➤ Fried chicken breast alone, with cheese melted over.
- ➤ Fried chicken breasts or tenders, sliced up, served mixed with cold diced tomatoes.
- ➤ Ham sandwich made of ham. 2 slices of ham, 1 slice of cheese and a bunch

of spinach. Squeeze the spinach and cheese between the two ham slices and eat.

➤ Beef hot dogs served over rice and sauerkraut. Mix in mustard and if you want your nose to run, sprinkle some cayenne in there.

➤ Pork ribs, baked. NO BBQ SAUCE

Beef has been for me the primary dinner. Ground grass-fed beef goes with just about everything. I've even mixed it into leftover chicken. Some suggestions:

➤ Fried packed together, cheese melted on at the end, like a burger. Separate with the spatula and eat.

➤ Fried all mashed and separated. Serve over rice or beans or spinach, or mix with greenbeans, NON-GMO corn, peas, diced tomatoes, mushrooms, sliced broccoli stalks... the combos are sort of limited to your imagination.

Do not over-brown your meat. Always cook beef well below medium heat. A slightly longer cook-time is preferable to activating the carcinogens using high heat.

➤ Spaghetti with organic tomato sauce. Be careful of your labels here. Your pasta is a wheat product. Buy only Italian wheat pasta. Use only organic tomatoes/sauces but watch for the addition of sugar. It doesn't need it. Mix in ground beef and a half cube of butter for a great pasta.

➤ Pasta with white sauce. Linguine, fettuccine, doesn't matter. I make the sauce melting a cube of butter in a pan. Add in ¼ cup of olive oil, ¼ cup of milk, 2 cloves of minced garlic, and about 1/3 pound of white non-hormone cheese. Slice up all that cheese and stir in, melting it all together. Dump the melted mess into your cooked pasta and season with basil and oregano. Some sea salt might be in order – let your taste buds decide. Mixing beef in this mixture is also extra good and chicken strips work, too. Don't be afraid to throw in some sautéed spinach when going chicken pasta.

But unfortunately, as good as some of this sounds, that's about the entirety of safe foods to eat.

Pizza? GM wheat crust, soy oil, canola oil, high fructose corn syrup or maltodextrin just in the bread, hormone-treated cheese mixed with MSG and soy lecithin, pepperoni with dextrose, flavorings and maltodextrin, tomato sauce packed with high fructose corn syrup, flavorings, colorings, sodium benzoate... Bah, I don't want to go on about it. Even the "best" pizza places use standard restaurant ingredients from the major suppliers. "Best" Pizza store owner: "I don't want the low grade MSG cheese, I want the high grade MSG cheese. We have standards, you know." "Best" does not mean healthy. I have yet to find a pizza using imported European wheat so we can be sure we're not getting GM wheat. **Forget pizza. Not even as a "treat."**

Chinese food? Do I need to bother? All restaurants, let me repeat that adjective "ALL", all restaurants are going to provide meals of varying quality using primarily the same suppliers. Soups? Canned. Salad dressings? Packaged or pre-bottled. Lasagnas? Prepared pasta made here in America from GM wheat. Salt? The chemical kind. Dinner rolls? GM wheat with soy oil.

Look, instead of filling this with finger-wag, let's just say that there is no safe restaurant, whether fast food or pricey, whether scumbag no t-shirt required to the hotty totty sniff sniff "that'll be seven hundred dollars for soup and a cracker" type places. Restaurants are pure poison – even the ones that claim they're vegan or healthy.

Next chapter will be about **condiments**. Mentioned some before but I should be more thorough.

CHAPTER 18

This chapter will be about **condiments** and **alcohol**.

It's so easy to grab a bottle of something and dump it on your food. But, they're almost all cancer.

Here are two safe ones:

Mustard – contains omega 3 fatty acids, calcium, phosphorous, magnesium and potassium. Mustard can improve your digestive function and help repair your digestive tract, reduces migraine frequency, increase metabolism and lower your blood pressure.

Goes good with beef. I often cook my meat in olive oil and a small pool of mustard. Gives it a rich flavor.

Olive oil – as a condiment, yes. Extra virgin olive oil is not only extremely beneficial to you but flavors your spinach salads and is good poured onto your leftover pasta or even your eggs. You want extra virgin – it is more expensive and should come in a dark bottle (light kills the nutrients). Extra virgin is

121

the first press of the olive, virgin is the second press. You're going to get your best nutritional value from extra virgin. Here's what olive oil does: protects against Alzheimers, breast cancer, bone loss and cardiovascular diseases. It is packed with antioxidants and is an anti-inflammatory food.

Here's a little rant. Many diet books will contain some truth and some common repetitions that do no one any good. One of my favorite "hates" is the word "**drizzle**." "Drizzle olive oil on this for a heart healthy... blah blah." Drizzle? Mind if I drizzle some drool into that nonsense? Drizzle. Take your olive oil and **pour it on**. Drizzling anything isn't getting you anywhere.

My other favorite "hate" word is "**helpings**." The insipid diet books tell you that you must eat 4 helpings of this a day, 9 helpings of that veggie, 14 helpings of the other veggie, a minimum 4 helpings of this fruit, 6 helpings of that other fruit, 11 helpings of another veggie, 12 helpings of whole wheat genetically modified garbage bread, 8 helpings of bran fiber to make you more constipated, 10 helpings of some dumb veggie like iceburg lettuce for some nutritionless empty calories. What a load. First, what the heck is a "helping?" Is it a handful? A forkful? A huge spoonful? A cup? 2 cups? 3 cups? A pinch? With big fingers or small?

What a bunch of crap. Even if a "helping" is very small, these diet books would have me eating *all day long* these fruits and veggies that I "must" have. I'd puke. Simple fact is, stop eating when you feel the hunger go away. Don't keep eating until you're stuffed.

Don't keep eating until you have cramps. Don't keep eating thinking you're going to have a food orgasm (I coined the term, "foodgasm"). There is no comfort food, there is only poison that feeds your addiction with chemical substances. Eating for "comfort" is another form of drug addiction.

When you begin to realize that food is just the fuel for the next toilet stool, then you begin to look at it less with love and more with utilitarian goals - "what can this food do for my body?" Not, "how can this food make me feel good?"

Onward.

BBQ Sauce: instant no-no. All full of high fructose corn syrup. MSGs and everything you must have to promote the fastest cancers possible.

Salad dressings: even "organic" salad dressing is full of organic soy (oh boy gosh!) and organic canola (more cancer please, pretty please). Ranch, thousand island, cheesy wonder dressings from some famous actor who knows nothing about healthy eating – yeah, all of those are just ways to feed you more poison.

Mayonnaise: I've been on a hunt high and low for a mayo that is only olive oil. There are a couple brands that scream at you "made with olive oil! But when you read the label, the primary ingredient is either canola or soy oil. A bullet to the head covered in genuine organic extra virgin olive oil is not good for you. Right? Right. So enough of that nonsense. Make your own mayonnaise using a stick blender and light olive oil[92]. Ingredients for homemade: 3 egg yolks, 3 tablespoons water, ½ squeezed lemon juice, 2 teaspoons of salt, 2 tablespoons of mustard, and 2 cups of light olive oil. Stick blender whips it up in less than thirty seconds and it tastes fantastic.

Bacon bits: no no no. Make your own. "Real" bacon bits might be made with real bacon, but are then covered coated sprayed and hosed down in MSGs and preservatives and who knows what else. Pick up a bottle of "REAL" bacon bits and see for yourself. Flavorings, spices, bleh. Fake Bacon Bits? Get real. Congealed MSG, snot, flavorings (MSG), some more snot, spices (MSG), and soy lecithin.

Steak sauce: No. All sugar with a hint of tomato paste. Plus some more MSG if you didn't get enough in the other crap "foods" being peddled.

Pickles: Generally no, but read your labels – it is possible to find pickles with only cucumber, vinegar, water and salt. Many pickles have "flavorings" and "spices" (more MSG in case you missed some).

Parmesan cheese: Has not been parmesan cheese for a long time. Genuine parmesan is super pricey. If you're buying it grated in a plastic shake bottle it is not parmesan cheese even though the label claims 100%. Kraft is being sued a second time over this labeling issue[93]. Grated parmesan cheese is stuffed full of MSGs the food manufacturers don't feel belong on the label because it was added during the formation of the cheese itself, rather than when grated.

Want a steak sauce? Try a blob of olive oil and some sea salt. Talk about delicious and juicy!

One last comment about food before I move on to alcohol.

Avoid the pastry aisle and just forget it exists. There is nothing healthy there, not the bran muffins, not the bagels, not the breakfast rolls, or cakes, or "fresh" cookies or any of it. I know, I've been there. All of it contains soy flour, soy oil or canola oil. All of it contains soy lecithin. Even the artisan bread made with whole wheat and olive oil with no soy or canola still uses genetically modified wheat and we know the gliadin in the wheat is responsible for the veritable explosion in stomach cancers, intestinal cancers, Irrititable Bowel Syndrome, and colon cancer. Don't do it.

These foods we grew up with are no longer foods. A Twinkie, perhaps faulted for being a bunch of bread and sugar, isn't bread and sugar anymore. The loaves of bread from 50 years ago might have been faulted for being bleached, but they were real bread, not genetically modified. So don't even try to pull the "oh I grew up on this so it can't be bad." It's not the same food. Not even close. And when you make an excuse to keep eating "just a little" of something because you like it, you are making an excuse to welcome the cancer, the pain, the genetic alterations to your own DNA, and a long, lingering painful death.

That's no finger-wag; it's the truth.

125

ALCOHOL. So much misinformation is floating around about booze that it is about as bad as politics.

On the one hand, a beer industry-paid article will claim beer is healthy and primarily water. Water can't be bad right? Hur hur.

Then we have the pot smokers who have decided to justify their own habit by talking all kinds of horror about alcohol and how it will destroy the world. Hur hur.

Throw in some religious people who claim that even a sip will cause an Exorcist style possession and you will burn in Hell.

Then there are some misinformed drinkers who claim alcohol has no glycemic impact and thus cannot possibly make you fat.

Before our heads start spinning and we start puking pea soup a'la Linda Blair, let's consider the science and ditch the hype. But first, to those who are religious, Jesus' first miracle was water to wine to keep the party going. I'm a Jesus-freak and can't help but shake my head that some think God must be limited by their own minds.

Alcohol can indeed make you fat with zero glycemic impact. Here's how.

To understand how this process occurs, let's examine the consumption of a 5 ounce glass of red wine. As the alcohol enters into digestion, it is split into two compounds: fat and acetate. The fat is taken through the bloodstream and stored wherever your body tends to deposit fat. The acetate is taken into the bloodstream and used as your primary energy fuel. **Read that last sentence again. The acetate is used as your primary energy fuel.** This means that rather than burning carbohydrates, protein, or fat as a fuel, your body relies on the acetate for energy. It completely stops burning anything else. Suddenly, you have a surplus of carbs, protein, and fat circulating in the body with nowhere to go. So where does it all end up? You guessed it... it's converted to fat and deposited on your waistline.

But wait, that's not all! As horrible as one drink can be, alcohol does something even more to sabotage your waistline. Alcohol consumption forces your body to produce cortisol, the hormone responsible for forcing your body to build more fatty tissues. It also reduces your testosterone levels, contributing even more to fat accumulation in estrogenic tissues[94].

Does this mean I swear off alcohol? Hell no and I'll tell you **one weird trick** that circumvents all of that: if you're going to drink, *do it on an empty stomach*. That carries its own dangers: overdrinking. Limit your intake to about half of what you used to drink because even half will get you trashed. However, in this way you avoid turning anything still in your stomach into fat, fat, and more fat.

What to drink, if you do? Avoid American alcohol unless it is made from potatoes. Most grains here in alcohol production are all GM – you don't want it in your system. American whiskey makes me gag with bile – a sure sign my body is telling me the product is no good. Scotch whisky is made without

GM grains, and thus safe to drink. Potato vodkas are good. Avoid beers as they are estrogenic. Be careful with gin as some gins use chemical flavorings that cause all sorts of neurotoxic nastiness.

Drink at night? Skip the meal and make sure you haven't eaten at least four hours prior to drinking and don't eat afterwards, either. I think you'll find that you begin to limit your drinking when you can't eat dinner.

Wine is a dicey choice. I prefer European wines over American due to our water contamination. But wine is a fine choice. A drink or two can lower blood pressure, lower your LDL cholesterol, and provide a few anti-oxidants in the mix that help fight cancer.

Don't be afraid of alcohol; but drink with limitation.

The end, and I hope this helps to germinate your own research, study and change in diet from "Please kill me" to "No, I want none of your diseases."

NOTES – REFERENCES

1: Journal of American Medicine, June, 2012 – as quoted in WebMD's News Archive, June 26, 2012

2: "Diabetes Strikes Younger and Younger" USA Today, November 13, 2007

3: "A History of Wheat Production in SD" October 29, 2012 as detailed at igrow.org/agronomy/wheat/looking-back-a-history-of-wheat-production-in-sd/

4: "Lose the Wheat, Lose the Weight" William Davis, MD

5: "The Economy in Fascist Italy" historylearningsite.co.uk

6: National Center for Biotechnology Information, "Demonstration of high opioid-like activity in isolated peptides from wheat gluten hydrolysates" Huebner FR, Lieberman KW, Rubino RP, Wall JS – as quoted 1984 Nov-Dec, www.ncbi.nlm.nih.gov/pubmed/6099562

7: USDA Food Pyramid, as shown at thetahealth.com/my-food-pyramid/

8: Professor Salman Hyder, as quoted in the article: "Celery May Help Kill Cancer" naturalnews.com/047369_cancer_prevention_celery_anti-tumor_activity.html

9: heart.org/HEARTORG/Conditions/Cholesterol/AboutCholesterol/Good-vs-Bad-Cholesterol_UCM_305561_Article.jsp

10: livestrong.com/article/283853-omega-3-in-eggs/

11: thechart.blogs.cnn.com/2012/08/15/is-eating-egg-yolks-as-bad-as-smoking/

12: meps.ahrq.gov/mepsweb/data_files/publications/st245/stat245.pdf

13: His financial advice didn't make the news. Later he formed Center for Health Transformation, a non-profit organization designed to morph HMOs into the larger medical conglomerates you see today. Bigger companies, bigger profits. Mission accomplished; he declared bankruptcy on the venture and shut it down in 2012.

14: drbenkim.com/articles-omega-3-fatty-acids.htm

15: ods.od.nih.gov/factsheets/Omega3Fatty AcidsandHealth-HealthProfessional/

16: www.optimal-heart-health.com
/omega_3.html

17: authoritynutrition.com/pastured-vs-omega-3-vs-conventional-eggs/

18: ethicalinvesting.com/monsanto/bgh.shtml

19: sott.net/article/162853-Your-Milk-on-Drugs-The-Dangers-of-rBGH-in-Dairy-Products

20: livestrong.com/article/446570-does-overheating-olive-oil-turn-it-to-trans-fat/

21: anh-usa.org/trans-fat-ban-not-what-it-appears/

22: As detailed by Doctor Akilah El, August 2011, docakilah.wordpress.com/2011/08/03/the-harmful-effects-of-canola-oil/

23: naturalnews.com/042054_organic_canola_oil_oxymoron_rapeseed.html

24: envirocancer.cornell.edu/Factsheet/Diet/fs37.hormones.cfm

25: biotech.iastate.edu/publications/biotech_info_series/Porcine_Somatotropin.html

26: legalzoom.com/articles/pig-patent-monsantos-efforts-to-claim-ownership

27: gmocompass.org/eng/database/ingredients/209.sweeteners.html

28:eatright.org/Public/content.aspx?id=6442463966

29: medical-dictionary.thefreedictionary.com/glucose

30: functionalps.com/blog/2012/03/19/ray-peat-phd-on-coconut-oil/

31: enenews.com/40000000-bq-of-iodine-131-in-a-single-bed-of-kelp-off-southern-california-amount-most-likely-larger

32: naturalnews.com/033716_sea_salt_health_benefits.html

33: asianews.it/index.php?l=en&art=11088

34: canada.com/health/health/4827169/story.html

35: foodconsumer.org/newsite/Safety/chemical/arsenic_antibiotics_1122110132.html

36: phys.org/news6067.html

37:coffeehabitat.com/2006/12/pesticides_used_2/

38: naturalnews.com/035595_Hershey_price_fixing_chocolate.html

39: non-gmoreport.com/articles/jun08/sugar_beet_industry_converts_to_gmo.php

40: healtharticles101.com/side-effects-of-too-much-estrogen/

41: chetday.com/bellyfat.htm

42: superfoods-scientific-research.com/superfoods/indole-3-carbinol-benefits.html

43: natural-homeremedies.com/vitamin-cure-for-depression/

44: Chemist Tony Xidis, PhD, (Kent State)

45: news.discovery.com/human/health/bpa-plastic-food-hormones-chemicals-110715.htm

46: medpagetoday.com/InfectiousDisease/PublicHealth/12767

47: proliberty.com/observer/20090608.htm

48: health-science.com/microwave_hazards.html

49: naturalnews.com/030651_microwave_cooking_cancer.html

50: articles.mercola.com/sites/articles
/archive/2010/05/18/microwave-hazards.aspx

51: wkyc.com/story/news/investigations
/2014/01/31/drinking-water-contamination-drugs-viagra/5087679/

52: digestivehealthguide.com/can-too-much-fiber-cause-constipation/

53: drweil.com/drw/u/WBL02077/Organic-Foods-Have-More-Antioxidants-Minerals.html

54: Chemtrails have been routinely denied by government and scoffers as the realm of tinfoil. But why are chemtrails included in legislation? This reminds me of the FEMA camp denials and the tinfoil labels thrown around about them. But the camps are real, are constantly mentioned in funding bills and can be seen directly in all states. Here is a link referencing legislation about chemtrails: theforbiddenknowledge.com/hardtruth/congressman_admits_chemtrails.htm

55: preventdisease.com/news/09/091509
_h1n1_chemtrail.shtml

56: jonrappoport.wordpress.com/2012/06/27
/how-swine-flu-was-invented/

57: articles.mercola.com/sites/articles
/archive/2013/05/13/mushroom-benefits.aspx

58: naturalnews.com/042996_sugar_ alternative_sweeteners_glycemic_index.html

59: thedoctorwithin.com/vitaminC/Ascorbic-Acid-Is-Not-Vitamin-C/

60: naturalnews.com/040147_vitamin_ c_ascorbic_acid_synthetic_vitamins.html#

61: webmd.com/diet/news/20120504/black-pepper-may-help-fight-fat

62: naturalnews.com/043054_curcumin _antioxidant_cancer_treatment.html

63: newmediaexplorer.org/chris/2007 /01/04/vitamin_c_sodium_benzoate_benzene_a_prov en_carcinogen.htm

64: livestrong.com/article/314356-the-harmful-side-effects-of-guar-gum/

65: naturalnews.com/044132_xanthan_ gum_mutated_corn_sugar_bacteria.html

66: naturalremediesthatwork.com/natural-remedies-for-heartburn/

67: livestrong.com/article/295738-olive-oil-for-acid-reflux/

68: Russel Blaylock, MD, website: blaylockreport.com/

69: foodmatters.tv/articles-1/the-dangers-of-msg

70: realfoodwholehealth.com/2011/05/excitotoxins-msg-and-hidden-names/

71: healthyanswers.com/nutrition/2009/04/the-untold-dangers-of-high-fructose-corn-syrup/

72: youtube.com/watch?v=QUCGn82l5u8

73: fsis.usda.gov/wps/portal/fsis/topics/international-affairs/us-codex-alimentarius

74: whale.to/b/damato.html

75: myfamilyhealth.webs.com/russiangmotests.htm

76: discovermagazine.com/2009/feb/22-very-tough-rat-big-risk-human-health

77: articles.mercola.com/sites/articles/archive/2010/09/18/soy-can-damage-your-health.aspx

78: westonaprice.org/health-topics/soy-infant-formula-birth-control-pills-for-babies/

79: Many sites claim that the skin doesn't absorb and scoff at the idea that our skin absorbs chemicals faster than ingestion. The following skeptic site showed several medical research references that proved our skin indeed does absorb far faster into the bloodstream than drinking or eating. Scoffing seems to be an industry now, but has no relation ro real science. Check here: skeptics.stackexchange.com /questions/5415/are-minerals-chemicals-absorbed-through-your-skin-during-bathing

80: undergroundhealth.com/sulfates-and-parabens-beware-of-the-potential-dangers/

81: Doctor Stephen Douglass, Doctor Russel Blaylock, and others

82: wnho.net/the_ecologist_aspartame _report.htm

83: articles.mercola.com/sites/articles /archive/2011/11/06/aspartame-most-dangerous-substance-added-to-food.aspx

84: riseearth.com/2013/03/dangers-of-aspartame-poisoning.html

85: globalhealingcenter.com/natural-health/concerned-about-aluminum-dangers/

86: dailymail.co.uk/news/article-2344845 /The-tomato-feared-200-YEARS-Europeans-called-poison-apple-thought-sinful-seductive.html

87: articles.mercola.com/sites/articles /archive/2013/11/27/toxic-perfume-chemicals.aspx

88: articles.mercola.com/sites/articles/
archive/2010/07/13/sodium-lauryl-sulfate.aspx

89: articles.mercola.com/sites/articles/
archive/2011/08/12/fluoride-and-the-brain-no-
margin-of-safety.aspx

90: articles.mercola.com/sites/articles/
archive/2011/10/17/aluminum-containing-
antiperspirants-contribute-breast-cancer.aspx

91: pakalertpress.com/2014/04/27/will-
humanity-survive-the-depopulation-agenda-of-the-
global-elite/

92: youtube.com/watch?v=GbPF_rLpd9o

93: chicagobusiness.com/article/20070205
/NEWS01/200023741/what-is-real-kraft-cheese

94: http://www.fitday.com/fitness-
articles/fitness/weight-loss/the-negative-weight-
affects-of-consuming-alcohol.html